Healing Hope

Healing Hope

A Journey

Lois V. Pike

iUniverse, Inc.
New York   Bloomington

Healing Hope

iUniverse books may be ordered through booksellers or by contacting:

iUniverse
1663 Liberty Drive
Bloomington, IN 47403
www.iuniverse.com
1-800-Authors (1-800-288-4677)

ISBN: 978-1-4401-0336-0 (pbk)
ISBN: 978-1-4401-0337-7 (ebk)

Library of Congress Control Number: 2008940905

Printed in the United States of America

Dedication:
This book and each word contained therein are dedicated to my loving husband, Wilbur, my children, step-children and our 6 beloved grandchildren:
Kendra, Ethan, Graham, Olivia, Eve and Glen.

To our beloved cat Sarah, who passed away earlier this Spring and to her sister cat Ella, who carries on. And also to our new "Big Boy" Tucker, who has come to join our family and provide us with his wonderful cat antics.

You have all provided me with the hope and sustinance with which to continue along my journey. HOPE is indeed the biggest word in my vocabulary.

Acknowledgements:

It would be remiss of me not to mention the following individuals. Each of them has been a most important aide and inspiration to the betterment of myself as a person living with chronic pain. I acknowledge their dedication to my belief in HOPE.

Aparna Oltikar, M.D.

James DeVanney, M.D.

John Carbon, D.O.

Sandy Deak – Dr's assistant

Diane Bray, A.P.R.N.

Amy Tobin – Massage Practitioner

*Dan McIntyre – President and CEO of The Charlotte Hungerford Hospital
All the nurses on the 2nd floor of CHH (you know who you are)*

Forward

"Most vagabonds I know
don't ever want to find the culprit
that remains the object of
their long relentless quest.

The obsession's in the chasing
and not the apprehending.
The pursuit perceived
can never be at rest."

Every time I get an inside view of the world of the chronic pain sufferer, not from a participant perspective (since I lack the pain credentials), but from an observer and caregiver view, I am reminded of the song lyric above. Often without ever having it stated overtly it becomes the mantra of the person for whom simply living anything like a "normal" life is a journey. It isn't the outcome of the journey, nor the destination that provides the incentive to not give in to the pain. It is simply being able to conduct the journey. To strive, to endeavor, to keep moving forward at virtually any pace is the goal. For the chronic pain sufferer the goal is not necessarily to win the game, it is simply to be able to play it at all.

So the pages that follow are from my bride, my partner and my constant inspiration to never give up, never give in to life's obstacles. Her message doesn't mean that you do not accept reality. The reality is whatever causes the pain. It IS real, whether it is visible or not. For the many people whom

I have seen Lois help with this journey, especially the "new" ones, the first step is to accept the reality of their pain source(s). She guides them to read, talk about and learn all they can about their pain source. In many cases, the source is immovable or incurable. It isn't temporary, rather a new permanent reality to learn to live with, like a relative you don't much like who has come to live with you. There is no available progress for the pain sufferer without accepting the reality of their situation.

But once that is accomplished well enough to serve as a reality anchor, the real journey begins and it is where the real trials start. Lois' first book "Embracing Life – Living With Chronic Pain" was about accepting the reality. Her next step is reflected well on the pages that follow. It is all related to choices. The pain source is reality, but the way one decides to deal with it is a matter of choice. Ultimately the choice is whether to renew your life journey or not.

When you decide to renew, the learning, dedication and fortitude needed will be very demanding and on some days just not possible. You will see of that in the following pages. But the obsession is in the chasing so on the next page you will find that you are well enough to travel and so you do. The speed, distance and destination are not the point. The point is about the fact that you are on the journey.

So the pages following are a sort of tour guide's diary of the chronic pain journey. These pages do not purport to be prescriptive for others, but to offer hope and inspiration. The writer's skill is evident in the words, but the strength purveyed through the words is the real gift for all of us, in pain or not.

Travel on!

Wilbur L. Pike III
August, 2008

The beginning of another new week
I ponder the healing process so far
And wonder if there is any real difference
Among all the illnesses there are

I contemplate what really works
Is it medicine or the gift of hope?
It's probably a little of both I think
Faith and prayer are the best ways to cope

I am filled with new hope for myself
For myself and other dear friends too
We are given these obstacles to overcome
Realizing that to ourselves we must be true

True beings sent from God are we
To follow the path He has chosen
For when we think that we are in charge
It is then we end up bitter and broken

A broken spirit is difficult to heal
For spirit is our true being
We must learn to hold onto our faith
And open our hearts in believing

That God truly has a plan for us
We need to pay closer attention
For when we listen to His soft whispers
It is then we quietly release all our tension

Another day of physical therapy is in store
Or will it be physical torture instead?
Some days that's what I think of it
While sorting it all out in my head

Today they let me walk on the treadmill
For an entire six minutes oh wow
I think they are simply amusing me
But they say this is progress somehow

If this is progress I'm just beginning to crawl
Oh how I yearn for the days
When I could do thirty pushups and then
Work out my body by lifting weights

But that was then and this is now
A fact that I must truly accept
My body has been ravaged by illness and now
I must move ahead without any regrets

Thank you dear God for this wonderful day
A day to improve myself and try
To simply accept what I have been given
And to stop asking the question "why"?

A day with no doctor's appointments at all
These days seem to be seldom and few
A day to relax and hold onto life
And be able to simply see it through

The pain monster is back and here to stay
The barometric pressure must be very low
My joints are all swollen and hurt so much
I must find a way to really let go

Let go and let God is my new motto to keep
It is much easier said than done
So I pray to God to give me the strength
To release the pain and simply move on

He is always there when I call to Him
What a wonderful God He is
He sends his angels who are our friends
To provide us with the necessary gifts

I am nervous because tomorrow is full
With surgery for my dear friend and brother
It is enough to send me into a full tailspin
But instead I pray to Our Father

A day of rest is finally here at last
To relax and pray as I see fit
I am thinking of all those deceased members
Of our family whose spirits with us remain lit

My mother is with me today as I pray
I can feel her presence very near
Somehow she is aware of our lives
The message she sends is very clear

She is smiling because she sees us together
My dear brother who has suffered much pain
Is here with me and my husband so loving
She does not have to worry ever again

Our family has changed over the past six months
And our living space is changing day by day
The new addition where my brother will live
Will be completed very soon we all pray

We are very happy to have him living so near
And to see his bright smile once again
God has sent His blessings to us all
And alleviated so much of our pain

Martin Luther King Day

As we celebrate the birth of Martin Luther King, Jr.
I am reminded of his wonderful speech and words
I had them mounted and framed for my husband
To hang in the office where he works

This is also the 19th anniversary of mom's passing
Quite coincidental for she was a librarian
She devoured books easily when she was alive
Our eldest grandchild is currently next in line

She reminds me so much of my late mother
If not a basketball, then a book in her hand
Mother has passed her love of books on no doubt
What a wonderful gift to have left behind

I find that I'm having a small "melt-down"
As I continue along with my day
I'm crying and praying at the same time
I must forge ahead and find my own way

So I ask for God's help to guide me again
And find peace on this memorable day
He guarantees us that He will send His help
If we simply pause and continue to pray

When at first I became so very ill
I sought out a therapist for some help
The pain was too much for me to bear
All I wanted was a clear way out

But that is not the message I received at all
I was taught instead how to manage the pain
I merely wanted to be rid of it for good
And for it never to come back again

What a fool I was to think in this manner
Of course the pain was from illness
But I was too proud to think I was sick
Somehow that made me feel so much less

Today I am blessed to visit with her once more
I am still learning and growing in my faith
I gift her with a bright set of prayer cards
That are each uplifting and filled with grace

She is very pleased with my growth thus far
And tells me so in her wonderful way
I will see her again in one month's time
As I leave her office I sing and pray

Today begins with a haircut, just a trim
With my friend Doug, the best in the business
He always knows and does just the right thing
And I leave with a big hug and a kiss

My brother is having his stitches removed
From the growth taken off last week
The nurse says the tissue was benign
And he is healing with very few small scars to see

Later this afternoon is physical therapy time
Once again I'm hoping to do a little bit more
I've finished the procedure of TENS followed with ice
And I am then lead out onto the gym floor

Oh boy I think, I wonder what I'll do?
I am put on the boring treadmill again
They allow me to raise the speed quite a bit
But only for eight minutes and then

I must stop for they don't want me to overdo
I could walk at least another half hour
I get off, head home and remember once more
Who really is in charge and has the power

The cats are all going to the Vet's office today
What a wild experience this is going to be
"Ella" and "Sarah" belong to us,
While "Miss Mary" my brother's makes three

My husband has a business appointment
And cannot join us for this joyful trip
Ella and Sarah sit by my side
And Miss Mary is joined to my brother at the hip

I am the one driving this happy day
We arrive after we travel so long
Miss Mary has entertained us all the way
Singing a not so very pleasant song

The treatments are completed and we drive home
The cats are all quiet as we drive
There is no one to greet us at the door
A great disappointment when we finally arrive

Later this evening we'll have a special guest
Our good friend and a blessing is our Joe
We will dine and catch up on many events
And celebrate his 30th birthday as we go!

Joe worked with me while I was at the Bank
And completed his law degree at night
He has been such a loyal and faithful friend
He is God's blessing to us, a true delight

The blizzard is over but I remain stunned
My pain has subsided and left me quite still
I long to stay warm under the covers
And simply look outside of the windowsill

A clean blanket of snow has left quite a sight
God's marvel of joy and splendor
I know that I'm forbidden to go outside
And so I quietly observe in complete wonder

I find that my energy has been depleted
Fighting the last two days filled with pain
I'm frightened again and in some sorrow
I pray to God to help me once again

I get up and read the morning paper
Looking to find some good news
The headlines are gloomy and so is the rest
I flip to the comic page hoping to be amused

Even the comics are laden with political satire
It seems we are the joke of the world
The war and horror stories fill each page
With new stories that everyday unfold

Dear God please help us to all find peace
In the entire world; no matter which country
The manner in which we conduct ourselves
Should be what matters most, not profit or money

A new week begins and I'm ready to run
Although I clearly know that's impossible
But the cleaning bug continues to bite
And so I do the little chores that I'm able

I start to finally dismantle the Christmas tree
And get every little thing in its right place
My brother helps me to pack it away
In what looks like a giant green suitcase

I then put the living room back in some order
It has been over crowded for quite some time
Now everything looks clean and properly placed
I feel proud just to follow the moderate line

Thank you dear God for allowing me to feel
A bit more complete as a woman of faith
Because when I'm down, I am really down
And when I'm up I cheer for the entire human race

I end up the day feeling peaceful and content
I've stuck to the moderate way and plan
I usually want to storm full speed ahead
Today I'm thankful for just who I am

The ground is all covered with newly fallen snow
I cocoon in the bed for the entire morning
It is such a beautiful sight to behold
I shall never get over such wonder and yearning

I see little children sledding down the street
In my mind as clearly as day
They are happy and having such great fun
And they wave to me along the way

God must have surely had children in mind
For most folks think snow is quite dreadful
Shoveling and clearing the driveways and walks
Grownups hardly ever seem to be cheerful

Easy for me to say as I stay warm inside
And never lift a shovel full of snow
It cheers me in ways I cannot describe
It is beauty beyond anything that I know

And so I read and write for the rest of the day
And wait for the men to arrive home
Laden down with groceries and whatever else
They enter the house with a groan

Thank you God for keeping me safe
Inside my warm little abode
Not having to go outside at all
Or help carry or have to unload

A very busy day is planned ahead for me
A visit to physical therapy this morning
And then a trip to the car dealership
To install my new rubber mat flooring

The therapy goes well and I am improving
But there remains quite a long way to go
Of course I want to see instant results
But I first must relearn how to crawl

Dear God it is really patience I need
Why is it so difficult to hold onto?
I manage to keep it for a few day's time
Then I lose hold of it, tho I never really intend to

I'm learning that I must pray for patience
Each and every day that I awake
For situation after situation I lose it again
And my health is what's really at stake

Thank you for the time to sit and relax
With others in the service's waiting room
I strike up a very pleasant conversation with someone
And then we are all gone much too soon

Yesterday was truly a great lesson for me
To be forced to sit still in the waiting room
I never once felt that this was taking too long
In fact the rest time let me plant a seed to bloom

On many topics currently breaking on the home-front
The woman I spoke with shared a lot of similar views
The television was blaring and she asked permission
To change the station and listen to the national news

I neglected to get her name as I left
Shame on me, I missed gaining a new friend
But her presence was indeed profound to me
We talked and a good ear she had to lend

Today I'm reflecting why we are put in such places
Certainly to be kind to and listen to others
There really could be peace in this world
If we treated each and everyone like a brother

Tonight we stayed home and talked for awhile
Husband and wife spending time together
We covered many a topic this evening
And went to bed feeling so much better

I sleep in late for I'm tired again
The temperature outside is bitter cold
My husband has gone ice fishing with his friends
I stay under the covers to warm my heart and soul

Finally I get up and come down the stairs
To find a hot burning woodstove so warm
It is comfortable inside our little farmhouse
I am delighted to stay inside all toasty and warm

Bert finally wakes and reminds me of
The errands we must run before noon
Good grief, I find myself hurrying again
The time to get rousing has come too soon

We head off to the bank and the post-office
And to drop off a few copies of my book
We arrive home long before Wilbur does
The time flies before I have a chance to look

Thank you dear God for rousing my spirit
Although my pain is pretty severe today
I am trying to take everything in stride
For moderation and patience I pray

This Sunday proves to be one busy day
I clean out my desk in the loft
By the time I am finished I have enough paper
To fill up a huge giant trough

I bring up an old tri-level table
To house my supplies and new printer
Everything seems to fit into place
I can now officially declare myself a "writer"

I am still in a lot of fibromyalgia pain
But I continue to move forward and press
I am pleased in the end with all the results
Why I work so hard is anyone's guess

I am surrounded with many words of wisdom
I thank God for providing me with this space
A space where I can be as creative as I'm able
This has indeed become a most sacred place

I pause for a bit and reflect on the day
I've finally been able to accomplish a big chore
And in so doing I find great satisfaction
Satisfaction is truly its own reward!

A new day begins and I am most grateful
A good time for pause and reflection
Yesterday left me quite shaken and startled
Now I must take even more precaution

I know that I am strong willed, even stubborn
But I want to make progress on this journey
I am going to class this evening to try
To move without too much exertion

I've been writing all day and now I must rest
If I'm ever to succeed in small steps tonight
Please God be patient with me and this yearning
To move in moderation with some foresight

I'm so happy to try to build up some strength
I am feeling like a small limp rag-doll
I know that if I pace myself slowly and right
I will have accomplished a small piece of my goal

And so I will go, put my feet up and rest
I will pray for Your insight and wisdom
I know that if I listen carefully to Your words
A new revelation for me will soon come

Last evening's adventure out was right on target
I actually felt the oxygen moving in my bones
I took very small steps, not pushing too hard
And was most happy to be missed by everyone

I worked very carefully, exercising every caution
And was glad that the movements were geared low
There are many new people attending this year
And the exercises were simplified and very slow

This allowed me to move around quite a bit
Which made me feel complete and filled with delight
It was as if a big load had been lifted from me
I thank God for I know He is always right

I arrived home and took a nice long hot shower
Bathing in my accomplishments for the day
I celebrated, having a cup of warm soothing tea
Watched some TV, smiling along as I pray

Today is a day to celebrate life indeed
Which reminds me of our annual celebration
We call it "Celebrate Life" in its tenth year now
I can hardly wait to send out the invitations!

The week is ending and on a good note
With no special plans except to lay low
Bert makes his monthly trip this afternnon
For the IV Drip of Zometa for his bones

Other than that we are all quite free
To busy ourselves or do nothing at all
I take my car to the car-wash for cleaning
It is so dirty from the previous snow fall

Whenever I enter or get out of my car
My clothes seem covered with chimney soot
I find this is most disturbing to the eye
Especially mine for I do not care for this look

I know that spring will arive in a few months
For I can see that the days are getting a bit longer
Oh how I anticipate the spell of warm weather
When we can see spring flowers in all of their splendor

The seed catalogues are arriving in the mail
We each choose many plants we admire a lot
Bert, the expert gardener helps us select
Which plants to grow in each garden plot

I know that the gardens will look terrific this year
Because of Bert's great gift of growing flowers
With his knowledge of plants and God's sunshine
The yard will look glorious in simply just a few hours

I arise quite early in the morning's sunlight
My mind is racing with ideas brand new
I come up to my little writing space
In the loft, which has quite a lovely view

I look around at the things on the wall
I have chosen such wise words of wisdom
And take a few minutes in which to capture
The meanings and where they each came from

"I am still learning" is at the very top
followed by the words of Emerson
"Let us be silent that we might hear
the whisper of God" resides near the bottom

Next in line is a favorite of mine
"All poetry is Prayer" is next to last
"Your Life is a Sacred Journey
and You are on the Path"

There are many more alongside of these
Some by Abraham Lincoln
His words are very meaningful to me
They are filled with great foresight and wisdom

Another week begins and I am inspired
With God all things are possible
We must have hope, love and faith
To receive His blessings so wonderful

I have just read that poetry begins
When childhood comes to an end
This explains why I've been writing
Since the grand old age of eleven

I was not aware at that time long ago
That my escape was in putting down words
The poetry then was very, very dark
I held many secrets unable to share

I wrote down things which were unbelievable
And somehow knew that I alone must bear
For who would believe a frightened young girl
Life was impossible for me to share

As for today and the world we live in now
Things are much different than before
I am truly blessed with words and music
To be able to compose a musical score

HONOR TO TERESA KELLY

It is my good friend Teresa's birthday today
She was named for St. Teresa, the little flower
At barely five feet one inch tall
She herself is a tiny, beautiful flower

She is one of the most loving and giving women
Always thinking of others before herself
She ran a group home for girls for many years
Providing shelter, love and a new life

I'm reminded how many people she has helped
To find meaning and purpose in their lives
For formerly abused children have little hope
Of ever reclaiming and living very useful lives

Many former residents return each year
To express their appreciation and love
For all of the many blessings received
From Teresa and from God above

She has been blessed with patience and grace
And has chosen the path of true giving
Her life is a model to emulate
And to prove that life is for living

I attended last evening's aerobics class
And found to my delight and surprise
That it wasn't that difficult for me at all
To join in almost every exercise

I paced myself, having learned to discern
That which I'm capable of and that which I'm not
To implement moderation and to not stretch beyond
Has been the lesson for me, which I think I've finally got

Knowing my limits has never stopped me before
I am experiencing the art of compromise
It is keeping me faithful in all aspects of life
Being true to myself with no disguise

Compromise has been a tough lesson to learn
Always thinking I could overcome with my mind
Any disability which has now become my life
And to treat myself more gently and kind

A strong will has always served me before
But strong willed does not mean being stubborn
Had I listened more closely with all of my heart
Patience would have been learned and reborn

Last evening's class was better than before
I'm feeling stronger and stronger each day
I know and adhere to the limits set for me
And use push-up time to meditate and pray

I enjoy a good long rest during the day
Knowing that I will be dancing tonight
As it turns out I dance nearly straight through
From seven thirty until almost midnight

What great fun we are having, each of us
To be so happy, loving and carefree
Although I had to hang up my tap shoes
I am able to dance softly with glee

The crabcakes I ate were second only to
The ones made in Baltimore Harbor
I enjoyed every single delicious morsel
And wished I could take some home to savor

I continue to be blessed with God's good grace
As I go about my regular daily living
I still experience much physical pain
But find that I am much more loving and giving

Valentine's Day has finally arrived
A day I very much look forward to
Not merely to express my love for my husband
But this year for my brother who is here too

We open our cards and presents with breakfast
What a happy threesome we make
We have each carefully chosen just the right gift
On that point there is clearly no mistake

I think of my dear mother this very day
It was supposed to be the day of my birth
But evidently I was in such a hurry to make
My grand entrance upon this earth

That I was born on December 30th instead
And quite a grand entrance I did make
Weighing in at under five pounds was I
There must have been some mistake

My father was serving in the Merchant Marines
And had to be called home just for me
I heard that it took a few days for him to arrive
He was delighted to have a daughter, waiting for him to see

"With God all things are possible"
I know this to be true
For I do believe in miracles
And have witnessed quite a few

Listen to the wind, how it howls
And the sky appears so gray
But look! It is not rain that falls
This is a soft white spray

Close inside I'm very warm
The fire glows ever so bright
The crispness of the covered ground
Glistens in the night

Through the glass I marvel
At this beautiful sight
It seems to possess some magic
It makes my heart feel light

Calling me there are things to do
And I know that I must go
But still I stand and marvel
At the new white fallen snow

A miracle indeed!

I am still learning albeit day by day
To listen more closely to the whisper of God
One must be still to hear those soft whispers
To be able to catch each and every wise word

Today I find myself asking for help
Not an easy thing for me to do
I must get rid of my pride indeed
And search from another point of view

I am only able to accomplish things
And form new ideas and thoughts
When I accept the gifts from God above
These gifts cannot simply be bought

Much more reading is available to me
Which will help me to discern and focus
On my small part in the world at large
And to continue to plant new seeds of hope

I met a new friend at aerobics class one night
Who is also suffering from bone disease
I was able to plant seeds of encouragement
When class ended, she and I both left quite pleased

I had dinner last night with two friends from work
And was reminded again about planting seeds
One never expects to ever hear of the results
From former acts of kindness and good deeds

A few years ago I was offered the opportunity
To cross-train a fellow worker of mine
She learned so quickly and proved such a help
Adding to the department with her ideas so fine

I was fortunate enough to spend one on one time
And before long her training was complete
But when I became ill and had to leave work
The department was looking a little bit bleak

She had returned to her former position by then
And was not at all satisfied to be there
When suddenly the opportunity presented itself
For someone qualified to fill my empty chair

She applied at once and was well assured
That she had the necessary skills to succeed
She thanked me last night for sharing with her
My knowledge, friendship and experience indeed!

One never really knows of the daily sowing we do
Or where those seeds will eventually lead
I was rewarded, blessed and delighted to learn
The results of my efforts and deeds

Thank you dear Lord for the chance to serve
In the manner which You have asked of me
I am filled with joy and quite overcome
To have opened doors by the faith living within me

I arise early and shower off the deep sleep
That took effect so early last evening
After breakfast, vitamins and my daily injection
I head off to a friend's for a day of visiting

She is delighted to see me and we talk for awhile
And then decide to go out and do some shopping
I still have some left over Christmas gift cards
Which leads us from store to store hopping

We find some great buys along our travels
My friend being the queen of shoes
We stop at the local footware store
And delight in what we finally choose

Then it is off to the local book-store
It's a favorite haunt for both ourselves
I marvel at all the many selections there are
And wonder if my book will ever see the shelves

We decide that we should do this more often
And stop for some coffee and a lovely chat
I purchase some wonderful new CD's
For me, books and music are where it's all at

Later this evening we are meeting good friends
My brother is excited to be going out
We each have a bite before we leave
To go dancing and visiting about

The weather is changing again, my body does tell
My knees are three times their size, what a blow
I turn on the weather station only to learn that
We are expecting eight more inches of snow

There are too many barom receptors in my body
I can forecast when the barometer is falling low
When there isn't enough pressure in the air
My joints swell, I ache and move very slow

I've learned a lot about weather and seasons
My body being the true measuring stick
When the barometric pressure is very high
I can easily move about lickety-split

Even in winter we are blessed with those days
We refer to them as the "Canadian Highs"
The air is clear and cold, but bright
One is motivated to spend time outside

We break around noon and head off to see
Our little friend play a game of basketball
The first half is exciting to watch every girl
The second half, they create too many fouls

As the clock runs out, they win the game
Although sloppily played, they are all grateful
We observe that they need to play more as a team
If they intend to make the playoff's at all

God gives us many different days to enjoy
There is meaning in each and every day
Some days are meant for rest and relaxation
But every one is a new opportunity to pray

It is President's Day, a holiday indeed
The day set aside to honor Washington and Lincoln
As a child I don't remember learning too much
About former presidents, especially Lincoln

I was raised in the South and learned more about
*Jefferson Davis, his ideas about slavery and living freely
He was indicted for treason and later released
The case against him dropped by influence of Horace Greely

He was the first and only President of
The Confederate States of America
He influenced President Franklin Pierce to sign
The Kansas-Nebraska Act increasing bitterness over slavery*

As an adult, I am fascinated by the words of Lincoln
So humble, rich in text and full of meaning
I surround myself with his words of wisdom
Which remind me that I am still learning

I believe him to be the truest President we've ever had
His regard always being for people and fairness to all
His faith carried him through many an ordeal
And he prayed daily for strength to carry out his call

He suffered many trials and tribulations in his day
His life was lived most honestly and faithfully
I would like to say that I live like Old Abe
But I must place trust in God more prayerfully

i

i From "Davis, Jefferson," Microsoft r Encarta r Online Encyclopedia 2005
http://encarta.msn c 1997-2005 Microsoft Corporation. All Rights Reserved

A friend sent this story to me recently and I wanted to share it with you. After searching the internet for the famous pianist, Ignace (Ignacy) Jan Paderewski, I found the piece to be fascinating, remarkable and totally inspirational:

*A mother, wishing to encourage her son's progress at the piano, bought tickets to a Paderewski performance. When the evening arrived, they found their seats near the front of the concert hall and eyed the majestic Steinway piano waiting on the stage. Soon the mother found a friend to talk to, and the boy slipped away. At eight o'clock, the lights in the auditorium began to dim, the spotlights came on, and only then did they notice the boy – up on the piano bench, innocently picking out "Twinkle Twinkle Little Star." His mother gasped, but before she could retrieve her son, the master appeared on the stage and quickly moved to the keyboard.

He whispered to the boy, "Don't quit. Keep playing." Leaning over, Paderewski reached down with his left hand and began filling in the bass part. Soon his right arm reached around the other side of the child and improvised a delightful obbligato. Together, the old master and the young novice held the audience mermerized.*

Perhaps that's the way it is with God. What we can accomplish on our own is hardly noteworthy. We try our best, but the results aren't always graceful flowing music. However, with the hand of the Master, our life's work can truly be beautiful. The next time you set out to accomplish great feats, listen carefully. You may hear the voice of the Master, whispering in your ear, "Don't quit. Keep playing."

May you feel His arms around you and know that His hands are there, helping you turn your feeble attempts into true masterpieces. Remember, God doesn't seem to call the equipped, rather, He equips the 'called'. May God bless you and be with you always!

ii

---

ii www.Paderewski.com Programs and Services – Solutions for Families
http://www.fww.org/progs.html

I continue to be struck by music once again
Listening to the wonderful voice of Josh Groban
Singing "You Raise Me Up", a truly marvelous tune
Being brought to tears from the beginning to the end

It is a beautiful melody about being down
and out with a heart very deeply burdened
And the solution is to simply wait quietly
Until God comes and speaks His words

It is so simplistic in its message to us
But we always want to know right now
The answers to all of our questions and fears
Without waiting patiently to learn how

To follow our hearts and listen for guidance
Which is always there available for us to hear
How I wish that I could be more patient with myself
And live more peacefully and not so much in fear

There is much to learn being quiet and still
Waiting silently and devoting time to pray
Healing hope is knowing that God will provide
The answer, which is usually just one prayer away

We traveled to the Town of Manchester today
To visit with good friends we've not seen for a while
I brought my friend a poem I'd written and framed
After reading it, she hugged me, and then cried outloud

Then she presented us with two prayer shawls
She knitted one for my brother and one for me
We're all so blessed to know and love each other
Later, we dined out for lunch and then had tea

Our friends are from Ireland and dear they are
They work and pray daily for those in need
No problem is ever too great to tackle
And with God's help, they always succeed

What faith and courage the two of them have
One Seventy Three, the other Seventy Five
They simply pray and place their trust in God
The reward being happy and truly alive

Their spirit is amazing to see and observe
And their works and deeds are such a wonder
What an inspirational message they send
Leaving all of us in awe and to ponder

A busy day of shopping is upon us
For new light fixtures and building trim
Brother Bert is too sore to go along this time
He leaves us to pick out the items for him

We have great success at the very first store
Although we still need to travel a distance by car
To order some new over-head lighting
For his new place is nearly completed thus far

How truly blessed we are to be able
To build on and have him next door
The painting is also nearly complete
The next thing is putting down the floor

We pray every day for one another's health
We are all battling some very great fights
With God on our side every moment of each day
We know that we will soon see some light

Thank you dear Lord for this opportunity to serve
We feel honored to do what You ask
When done with great love and humility
Nothing You ask is too difficult a task

I am writing a thank you to my dear granddaughter
For the lovely gift she presented to me yesterday
She hand-made a pillow in Home-Ec class
And wrote a lovely message on the back just to say

"Hey, Lil Grammy, I made you this cute pillow in Home-Ec
because I know just how much you love the UCONN team.
I miss you so much, but now when you see this pillow,
You can think about your favorite team and me!!"

Now I ask you, what greater love could there be
Between grandparents and their devoted grandchildren?
Never having had any grandparents to call my own
I am humbled to tears as I read this again and again

What a gift from God she is and the pillow too
Something to cherish and hold for a lifetime
She knows that I'm ill and often in pain
But she always manages to let her light shine!

I am blessed with our children and their children too
To have them to share is a delight sent from God
It is a reward somehow for putting in all those years
This love is ever so safe, like peas close together in a pod

Today marks the end of a month of the year
I'm feeling uplifted in spite of the snow
For Spring is now just around the corner
Just waiting to let her lush soft green show

I think our lives are much like the seasons
In wintertime we feel the need to cocoon
And then a brand new season arrives
Welcoming us with soft colored blooms

I know that my pain will be lessened a bit
I will act and feel much more alive
For even when those spring showers come
I will still want to spend time outside

I can't wait to see the soft flowers of spring
Which we planted last fall in the garden
It's a miracle to see them peep their little heads
From beneath ground previously frozen and hardened

I know how the past winter was for me
Afraid to go out and perhaps take a fall
This bone disease is very risky business
When one has previously broken many bones

But alas, the wintry days are coming to an end
And healing hope is once again high in the air
Healing and hope are indeed on my list
And to that end I bow my head in prayer

So much for spring, we are having a "Noreaster"
A giant storm depositing fifteen inches of snow
March in New England is a "trickster" month for all
Turning over the calendar there are pictures that glow

With the promise of Spring and Easter bunnies
Of green grass, baskets and glorious straw hats
Looking outside is like viewing a foreign country
In winter, like Austria's snow covered mountain caps

We gather around the wood-stove for warming
And have coffee and tea and toast to eat
There is no place to go, the roads are all covered
And so we take this time off and call it a retreat

Hope is still burning in my spirit today
Along with the stiffness and pain
But soon these snow showers will fade away
And we'll feel Spring's soft healing rain

Another day to give thanks and prayer
To remember that God is in charge
Disruptions in our lives are difficult to deal with
We need to learn to live life fully at large

To take advantage of each and every day
No matter the disappointments they may bring
We will fully appreciate as the seasons change
When at long last we can finally see Spring!

This day of balance seems to be a test of wills
Not everything is equal in time for me
Fibromyalgia has again reared its ugly head
I want to get up, move around and be free

The pain manifests itself in brand new places
This catches me quite off-guard and by surprise
The need for total rest in bed presents itself
I am disappointed, this is not where my vision lies

Looking and feeling pretty lousy I am
I can barely manage to just function
Another day set aside to relax and pray
I would much rather be in motion

It is a chance to ponder the future picture
And face my own fears straight on
After all this is merely one day of my life
I focus on my purpose and somehow carry on

I listen to soft music which lessens the pain
My body calms down and becomes still
Taking my meds is still a problem for me
I'm reminded sternly to follow God's will

Empowerment comes from placing my trust
In God and my long living faith
I wrap myself up in my new Prayer-Shawl
And lay open to receive God's grace

I awake feeling totally rested and alert
As I think about last evening's conference
Imagine a catalogue company that gives something back
To communities via their program "Making a Difference"

It seems that we all are blessed to know
People whose mission statement is for others first
I am lucky indeed to have heard these women
Speak of their visions and passions and who thirst

To assist other women in many different walks of life
Sharing their meaning, purpose and direction
Giving back some of their good fortune and blessings
To encourage young women who are still searching

I am overjoyed knowing what path lies ahead
And am quite clear about my purpose and vision
It is to write and encourage women everywhere
To live life to the fullest, without over extension and exertion

For there is healing hope living in each of us
Which needs to be let out and spread around
To provide vision and relief for those who suffer
And are in need of finding a higher ground

God is always there bestowing His blessings
And grace to those who remain open
To accept each day and that which it offers
There can ultimately be no greater plan

A bright new morning sun beckons to me
I move as my spirit, being replenished, is high
I manage some chores, changing bed linens and towels
At long last, there is energy to claim as mine

I eat a good breakfast and take my morning meds
And administer my daily shot in my thigh
My joints are aching, the barometer must be falling
I look up questioningly towards the sky

Not too soon after the sun begins to fade
And here come the clouds so dark and gray
Now it is beginning to snow heavily
God's blessing, a soft white spray

Spaghetti sauce is simmering on the wood-stove
Filling the air with fragrance and appeal
I dare not go down to taste one tiny bit
I wish to savor the sauce for our evening meal

What a wonderful day, warm and toasty inside
With the wood-stove being used for cooking
Smiling and glancing outside at the miracle
It is God's gift to us, free for the looking

I cherish these days with my husband and brother
Together we are a three-some family
We have seen much healing these past six months
We rejoice and count our blessings happily

A busy day begins for all three of us
My brother has two Doctor visits to make
One at the Cancer Center for his monthly IV- drip
The other his every three month shot to take

The day progresses just fine and dandy
Until we arrive back home at long last
Wilbur has decided to stain the 16 ft rafters
The ladder falls and we hear an enormous crash

We go rushing inside to see what happened
My brother thinks someone has driven a car into the house
We find that Wilbur is laying quite still on the floor
He has fallen and lays very quiet as a mouse

We check him over completely and ask
Do you think you should be seen at the hospital?
He is able to move all of his joints and replies
That he seems only to be very badly rattled

Now here is a genuine miracle if ever
To ride 16 feet down on a ladder
We tell him that if he wants to go for a ride
Many parks provide rides so much cheaper

God has protected our loved one again
The damage could have been so much greater
We are grateful to God just one more time
Healing Hope and prayer really do matter

There is not only snow but a blizzard outside
With winds over 50 miles per hour
We cannot see our barn across the street
This storm has great umph and power

It continues to blow with such a force
It is a bit frightening to look at it
I'm afraid to venture outside today
Lest I be blown completely to bits

We have the wood-stove burning on high
To ensure that we remain safe and warm
There is a marked difference between outside
And the inside warm cozyness and calm

Dinner is prepared on the old gas viking stove
When immediately the lights go out for the night
We listen to our favorite basketball game
Via a battery powered radio with delight

The power remains off for merely 3 hours
This is a relatively short time for us to say
For living out here in the country this far
We can be without power for at least 3 full days

It takes a great deal of "Yankee Ingenuity"
To survive in the depths of winter
And God is always there by our sides
To provide His wisdom if we only surrender

The sun has finally broken though the skies
Although the temperature remains bitter cold
Thankfully we have a house to live in
God is clearly protecting His fold

We all remain busy at our computers today
From all over the house the clicking comes
With messages and proofs for me to review
Sometime very late in the day, I finally succomb

I have proofed and reviewed as long as I can
Ensuring that there are no more corrections to make
My eyes are tired and so also are my fingers
It is now time to take that long overdue break

Bert and I have Chinese take-out for dinner
While Wilbur joins his friendly Wednesday group
Since he is not able to participate in the game
He joins them for pizza and a laughing hoot

I am watching "Doc" on PAX TV
I love this station and all it represents
There are always exceptional morals and values
Revealed in each and every episode's events

My prayer tonight is for continued healing
For myself and others who are in pain
I ask God to forgive any residual anger
To cling tightly to hope and all there is to gain

This day begin slowly, quite lazily it seems
Though we have many things to achieve
I am going for my hair to be trimmed
And then to Bert's storage place to retrieve

The music that is needed for the Memorial Mass
To celebrate the life of our friend's dear father
I need also to get my 12 string guitar restrung
My playing has lapsed, I remember and then ponder

I'm familiar with the selections which have been chosen
I simply need to put my hands on the strings
My brother will be playing the grande pipe organ
While our entire music group sings

This night I plan to return to aerobics class
It seems like I'm always starting over
But I'm learning to field and accept the setbacks
While God above watches over me and hovers

I am feeling profoundly inspired this day
To reach out and be one with the world
I have great hopes to conquer my pain
And to share my experiences through words

My wish is for everyone everwhere
To keep hope alive in their hearts
To embrace hope ever so tightly now
That it becomes one of our living parts

We had planned to travel 53 miles to church today
To look for some much needed music for the organ
But alas, it is snowing quite heavily once again
This is the 4th snowstorm since the snows began

Last night I attended my low impact aerobic class
And my body is still slowly recovering
It is speaking to me in many new ways
Perhaps that is why it is snowing

God telling me to take a well deserved rest
When I want to be traveling out and about
I reluctantly yield to His message at last
Not pretending, my face wears a pout

I generally don't like receiving gifts
I much prefer the role of the giver
I wanted so much to drive across state
And to be able to assist my dear brother

I find myself catching up on some mail
And sending along some good wishes
To many folks who have been so gracious
Some helping with housework and dishes

It is time now for me to take my daily meds
Along with the dreaded Forteo shot
Motivation eludes me as I sit here
But I remember to offer thanks to God

I find myself humbled to tears this day
God is clearly using my written pages
To help another woman break through her grief
And the constant pain she has lived with for ages

She is reading my draft of "Embracing Life"
And finding new meaning in her life
She has opened a notebook to record her thoughts
Reflecting on her chronic pain and strife

To know that my words have moved another
And help deal with the matters at hand
Are reward enough for me to continue
On the path that is clearly God's plan

If only one person receives some benefit
From reading the book I have carefully written
Then I feel as if I have accomplished a great feat
I thank God for the gift which He has given

I speak with both she and her husband so kind
He is elated that she is finally gotten into a space
Reading a book that has meaning directed at her
We all rejoice for she relates and is now in a better place

Last evening out proved to be a fabulous time
We went to hear Linda Eder in concert live
She has the most amazing voice – a 4 octave range
We sat mesmerized listening to her music divine

When I awoke this morning ever so early
I was surprised that I hadn't slept until noon
I took my coffee and the newspaper upstairs
And fell back to sleep until well past noon

Since the concert was 1 ½ hours drive each way
We arrived home somewhere late after midnight
I realize now I had not gotten quite enough sleep
Which is why I slept through the morning's light

Upon rising the second time, we set about doing chores
Moving some furniture about from room to room
To make a fresh appearance and clean the stale
Significantly changing the look of our home

My brother will be moving into the addition soon
And clearing out the over-crowded space
I am looking forward to the annual spring cleaning
Most people I know think that I'm crazed

Spring cleaning is like a purification act
It is motivation to renew my faith and hope
It is cleansing, providing me with God's good grace
To make the best of the things I love most

It is off to the tax man early this morning
To supply him with all of our records
This has been a most difficult year
Accounting for all of our medical records

My brother and I also sold our house
That which we owned jointly together
The funds are being used to fund the addition
And soon he will move in, much to his great pleasure

It is a bright day outside with skies of azure
An amazing day after all the previous snow
For in the middle of March we all hope to see
Some green grass with yellow daffodils for show

Here in New England we must wait until April
To see and hear the sights, which we love
Even in April we can experience some snow
And we look hopefully with faith to God above

We accept whatever He sends to us
And since Easter comes very early this year
I'm afraid the children will be hunting for eggs
Deeply burried in the snow for them here

No sign of yet that Spring will be arriving
Anytime soon, I'm so sorry to say
Please dear Lord hear our many prayers
And send Spring along now any day

Mother Teresa has spoken many beautiful quotes
This certainly is one of my favorites:

"I have found the paradox that if I love until it hurts
then there is no hurt, but only more love"

I read this paradox every single morning
It hangs on the corkboard next to my desk
I can only imagine what she is referring to
As I ponder the works that God asks

We are called upon to show more kindness
Each and every single solitary day
And although I try my best to comply
Some days I shamefully stray

Today was a day to reflect and pause
I chose to not share much of myself
And put my needs before many others
Gracious was clearly not how I felt

Later in the day we drove to see our grandson
And took him to dinner to finally celebrate
The pleasure returned just watching him
Open his gifts and seeing him feeling so great

The lesson is once again presented to me
Sharing myself is being asked for by God
I so much want to leave the door wide open
For healing hope to enter, I bow and humbly nod

St. Patrick's day is here to greet us again
Our many Irish friends rejoice in their hearts
Being of Italian and Scottish descent
Celebrating of the green is separate and apart

There are green shamrocks and green hats
And even green bagels and green beer
St. Paddy's day is one big celebration
Everyone seems to be of good cheer

What a fun day placed in the middle of March
While we all await Spring's natural color of green
For now the snow isn't perceived as a miracle anymore
We are looking for the soft breezes and air so clean

Later today we will travel far to church
To practice music for Saturday's Memorial Mass
Celebrating the life of our dear friend's father
Whose life here on earth has recently passed

We will be twelve voices singing together
The number twelve as in the Apostles
Working together to create a joyful noise
With God, anything is truly possible

I feel very positive about this endeavor
It will be accomplished with such great love
It is said that singing is praying twice
I hope we sound like sweet angels from above

Imagine my surprise when opening my mail
To learn that my first book had been published
Although it took one solid year to write
I am enjoying it and every word written I relish

To be able to respond to my being dis-abled
Which is not the way I think of myself at all
Yes, I do have limited physical ability
Thus I am responding to a much greater call

Healing hope has become a part of my being
It is an internal organ living within me
It started out small, then grew very large
And remains such a powerful source of energy

If I make just one person think differently
About their physical or emotional pain
Then I know that I will have achieved success
For that is my ultimate goal to gain

There are many out there who believe in me
And all that my writing has to tell
With the help of their unwavering support
I continue on this mission quite well

God continues to bless us all
Something I never lose sight of
I thank Him every day and night
And accept His blessings from above

We are all up early this very special morning
We will travel to Manchester for our friend
To sing in celebration the life of her dad
Whose time on earth has come to its end

The church is filled almost to capacity
With folks some known and others not
But we are here to sing our very best
To comfort the family, they number a lot

We sing with such glee, it almost seems odd
This is a Memorial Service we're singing
But our voices are raised in true celebration
We are remembering the life of another human being

The service is over and we receive applause
We are humbled and amazed at the same time
We would like to continue singing once a month
The spirit and music are simply divine

Everyone is invited downstairs to enjoy
Good food, company and most of all sharing
We are each of us filled with overflowing joy
As we receive compliments on our music and caring

We leave to come home after an hour of visiting
With the family and friends so dear
I secretly wish that we could continue
To sing straight throughout the coming year

Another new week begins for us at last
It is still March; however, and very overcast
I've always heard that March comes in like a lion
And leaves like a lamb, someone must be lying

The temperature is falling, it is getting so cold
And today I am feeling quite antique and old
The barometer is dropping at such a fast rate
I'm certain of what's in store, I can predict my own fate

But this time I try a new way to deal with it
Prayer, hope and rest to which I now must commit
This is helping to take my mind off the pain
I am relentless, I will try this again and again

I head out the door with promotional items in hand
It is off to the office store I drive until I land
Presenting these items to be copied on card-stock
I am feeling quite elated as I drive down the block

Tomorrow I will pick up posters, cards and bookmarks
These represent the new writing venture, which I have started
My spirit is lifted by these new books which I write
With the goal of helping others to reach for new heights

I am blessed beyond reason to have found at long last
The true calling for me of which Spirit has asked
To simply recount my experiences on paper to read
That others may be helped in their time of need

A most significant day in my life has begun
I am moving ahead with my project as if somehow seduced
I pick up my items, which were dropped off yesterday
And marvel at how clearly and well they were reproduced

I am sparkling and smiling as I drive next to the fabric store
To purchase some material to make curtains for my brother
He'll be moving into the addition this Saturday afternoon
My love for him is magnificant, it is truly like no other

We are blessed to have him here with the family
He has become one with us and he loves it out here
In the quiet countryside, without all the noise
Away from the big city, where he can finally heal

We have gotten to know him as funny and clever
And of course as musician and gardener so well
We see a side of him, which was previously hidden
He is now free to let his wisdom ring out clear as a bell

This brother of mine, whom we thought would be dead
Has been resurrected to life, what a gift to us all
God must have plans left for him here on this earth
We rejoice as we remember last summer and fall

Cancer had taken a solid grip on his life
As he lay motionless in bed for a very long time
But, alas he came out to our little farmhouse
Treated by the best doctors and hospital in town

I have received more clarification than I could have asked for
To know that I'm doing the work I was placed on earth for
To assist other people dealing with chronic pain or worse
To provide healing hope when all else seems lost or cursed

This is God's work, I'm simply along for the ride
To withstand the raising and lowering of the tide
This is a metaphor worth giving time to heed
When one is living with pain and so many other needs

To dismiss or forget that life moves like the tide
Is like ignoring that which lives within us deep inside
We ride the waves of life, hoping to rise above
And capture, somewhere along the way, a thing called love

It is different for each of us, that is for certain
Life can end abruptly, closing the curtain
But what is left behind is our own legacy
Were we fair and honest to people other than we?

I have been blessed by both disease and pain
For through it I have fought hard my life to regain
If adversity had never been placed at my door
I may have chosen many other folks to ignore

But I have been graced by God and been chosen
To reveal His hope, His healing and wisdom
I will ever be changed by this chance in my life
To grab opportunity and choose hope over strife

The subject today is about maintaining proper balance
A very tricky thing for all who are called
I'm thinking of an olympic gymnast for instance
Knowing exactly where to place those feet to prevent a fall

It takes years of practice and I am still learning
When to push forward and when to pull back
The very art of maintaining pure balance
Is a challenge, even for those who have the knack

We try ever so hard to keep from burning out
There must be time for work, prayer and play
How seldom do we in fact find the time?
And how do we justify that all in one day?

How do we accomplish true balance at all?
We must all try harder with each day granted
Responding differently to each separate challenge
To learn in fact, to bloom where we are planted

A few nights ago, while working in class
We were all doing planking, a most difficult move
I found myself distracted by the groans around me
And focused on prayer, which allowed me to use

This most sacred time set apart just for me
By praying I no longer heard all the chatter
I was able to sustain the position much longer
Which was my intention and what really mattered

Easter Sunday arrives quite early this year
I always try to figure the formula out
It's the first Sunday after the First Full Moon
Following the Vernal Equinox

This year it arrives early in the season
We still have a mountain of snow on the ground
While other parts of the state are finally seeing
Flowers peeping through the soft new ground

But we in the northwest corner of the state
Will have to suffer with cold another few weeks
Hopefully the winter snow has come to an end
And soon we will see crocuses start to peep

Although spring arrives later in this part of the state
When it finally arrives, it manifests itself quite fast
How I look forward to those yellow sprigs of forsythia
Announcing that spring is really here at long last

Today I rest for almost the entire day long
My joints remain swollen and very sore
Probably due to yesterday's work overdone
But my spirit is flying and ready to soar

Bert is spending some time in his new place
Along with his beloved cat "Miss Mary"
How happy he is to have a new home at last
He is singing brightly like a trained canary

Thank you dear Lord for this day to relax
And celebrate Your rising from the dead
I feel like my spirit has risen from the ashes
And to You I pray and lower my head

The swelling has subsided now in my wobbly knees
And I am feeling much relieved, my faith has been restored
We travel over one hour distance to see my favorite Doc
He delivers his advise to us and sends me down the hall

Oh boy, more blood to draw, no wonder I'm anemic
He is testing for Lyme Disease and other things no doubt
He listens very carefully to what we have to say
And tells me not to push too hard, as we are heading out

Oh how I wish there were some magic elixir
To pass around to all those suffering in pain
But we must each of us find our own way
To happiness and live within a laid out plan

The weather today is warm and sunny
The barometer is clearly on the rise
For the air is clear, crisp and clean
To me this comes as no big surprise

Healing Hope is arriving just like Spring
With warm dry weather to provide hope
I can feel it deep down in my bones
In my mind, I can almost feel myself float

The birds are softly chirping their song
Although there remains quite a bit of snow
God sends them to remind us I'm sure, that
Before too long a-gardening we will go!

The very last day of March is finally here
And I am most happy to see her go
For April will now shine her glowing face
And melt away the last bit of snow

The sun has beckoned to me this morning
How cheerful and delightful are the morning rays
It awakens my faith and hope once more
My child-like self wants to run and play

Spring does awaken our hearts and spirits
From the long and cold hard winter
We see God's brightness outside the door
And invite her to abide in us, to freely enter

The trees are spreading their branches wide
As people embracing life and opening up their souls
To breathe in every tiny breath of Spring
While we gently let our hearts unfold

What a glorious day God has provided
To lift the solemnity and glum
Which previously had taken up residence
In my heart, but which now has finally flown

I'm amazed at the difference one day makes
When so diminished can be the pain
It proves to me that prayer is the elixir
And Healing Hope has returned again

April has arrived with the entire world watching
As the health of the Pope continues to fail
But we are concerned about our dearest friend Don
Who lies home in a hospital bed complete with rails

We know that he will be passing on very soon
And we have all wept the entire week long
He fought such a difficult battle with lung cancer
For someone who was once so vibrant and strong

We feel his presence this morning in our room
He is passing through saying his last goodbye's
And thanking us for providing such joy in his life
Knowing and loving him so long proved to be our prize

I think of him all throughout the day
And pray for him, his family and lovely wife
They remain the best of friends themselves
His passing will somehow ease his pain and strife

God is blessing each of us right now
With His undying grace and love
Don grows much weaker during the day
Please God, send Your angels from above

I pray tonight that Don will finally let go
And surrender to a quick, peaceful passing
My tears continue to flow in a steady stream
I trust in God's love which is everlasting

We receive the call very early this morning
Don's fight on earth has come to an end
I find that I'm astonished with my own feelings
I am peaceful and calm at the passing of my friend

We are asked to select and play the music
That will be sung at his funeral service
I put this aside for later in the day
I must think very carefully during this process

My wonderful friend arrives at about 10:30
For our previously planned day of going out
This proves to be an excellent diversion
For there are too many things to think about

We head out the door for a day of shopping
And enjoy oursleves and finally break for lunch-time
We find we are both ravenous at this late hour
We make our selections, the food is simply divine

We stop one more time before we head home
The store is filled with lovely items reflecting spring
I choose two forsythia wreaths for the front doors
One for us and one for my brother when his doorbell rings

We arrive home at long last, laden with packages
For we have made a day of being together
Everyone is delighted with the gifts they receive
Now we really need a change in the weather

The clocks have been moved forward, we arise too early
We wait before making the necessary phone calls
To see who will be available to rehearse and to sing
There will be ten of us this time in all

Helen has asked for happy and peppy music
This will be a celebration of life and love
Bert and I are busy, making wonderful selections
To send Don off to his heavenly home above

The rest of this day consists of answering e-mails
And making notes about the trying days to come
I gain a new perspective concerning life and death
Life as we know it on earth is finally done

But now we will have our own guardian angel
Watching out for each of us, his friends
Our lives continue and we press on with living
I'm aware now that life never really ends

I have lost many friends and relatives before
There is something quite different this time
It appears as a brand new revelation to me
That life is always on a continuum line

Thank you dear God for this new teaching
It has brought me such comfort and calm
When I take the time to sit quietly and listen
Your words transform me like a soothing balm

Today we will travel to Manchester again
The trips are beginning to tire me out
But this day we will attend the wake for "Uncle Don"
And then head home for a well needed time-out

There are hundreds of folks in attendance this afternoon
I can only imagine what the evening hours will bring
The family seems to be holding up quite well
And I prepare myself for tomorrow when we will sing

It is a warm, sunny and bright spring day today
People don't have to wait outside in the cold
The lines wrap around the building in circles
There are so many folks in "Uncle Don's" fold

We stay for close to an hour and one-half
Before bidding our final fond farewells
I am drawn to this family and don't want to leave
But we must, to make room for the others as well

We drive home silently, I find myself reflecting
On all that Don has meant to me throughout our lives
He was Mentor, Dad and even Grandfather
To my little family and to others, no surprise

Thank you dear Lord for the blessings you bestow
We now have our own Guardian Angel above
Don can now watch over each of us in turn
While sending down Your everlasting love

We all arise quite early with different places to go
Wilbur has a conference scheduled for the entire day
Bert and I travel back to Manchester this morning
Finding ourselves in rush hour traffic along the way

We finally arrive at church in plenty of time
To tune up and lay out all the music, which is long
We are delighted to find more people than we planned
Who are willing to help us out with the singing in song

This is definitely a day to remember forever
Fr. Clancy considers Uncle Don a true Apostle
And relates that to the entire congregation
What a glorious send off, to sing is nearly impossible

But sing out we do with our hearts filled with spirit
We also want the congregation to know how we feel
The music is a fabulous tribute to Uncle Don
The family and congregation are all moved to tears

We hold each other up though we all want to sob
We cannot allow for this emotion to take over now
For we have a job to participate and complete
To end the service with a great big WOW

Helen (Don's wife) applauds at the end
And invites the congregation to join in with her
She is beaming and we can feel Uncle Don's smile also
Thank you God for this opportunity to once again serve

I retired to bed much earlier last evening
And counted the blessings for the day
I was unable to see them clearly yesterday
But then God always shows us the way

Late in the afternoon, our friend and neighbor, Bob
Responded to the call in his heart
He knocked at the door with a present for me
He gifted me with "The Power of Intention" by Wayne Dwyer

Something told him that my spirit was down
And he actually stopped in the middle of his work
To come, sit and visit with me for awhile
He trusted in God's prodding and knew that I was hurt

I am humbled and amazed at how God's spirit works
Or rather, how true friends listen and respond
What if we all listened deep within our hearts
And acted upon the words from beyond?

Bob reminded me the words lie within each of us
We simply need to be silent to hear them
I agreed with that thought and knew I needed rest
And quiet time to draw back inside to regain them

Thank you dear Lord for another time-out
To reflect on Your words living within me
I frequently seem to forget to take rest time
And sit quietly and allow You to replenish me

Last evening we dined at the home of good friends
Whom we have not seen in a few years time
It was most powerful to re-connect once again
The entire evening seemed to have quickly flown by

Linda had become my dear friend and tenant
Some twenty odd years long ago
She is lovely and beautiful at the same time
Her spirit shines through wherever she goes

We met her new beau, Spero is his name
A fine gentleman in his own right
With a wit as quick as old Mark Twain himself
He entertained us for most of the night

What blessings we have in friends who care
Whether we see them often or seldom
It is always like meeting for the very first time
We immediately all felt welcome

I had so much to share that I could barely shut up
When I realized it was time to depart
I'll try to listen more and speak much less
And heed the message deep within my heart

I've a grand list of things to accomplish
And marketing is at the top of the list
There are so many calls that I must make
To book stores, newspapers, you get the gist

My book order arrived late last week
Now I must make those important connections
To glean bit by bit those who are truly interested
And set up meeting times for the book's inspection

I've already met with the good folks at the bank
And followed up on some of their leads
Reaching out is the easy part for me
I want to touch all those readers who have needs

And so as the day moves peacefully along
I find my work much easier than I expected
Everyone I call seems genuinely intrigued
By the content and poetry, which are so connected

I stop to thank God for His many gifts bestowed
Upon me, my family and many good friends
I continue on with my numerous phone calls
As the day winds down towards its end

Now it is time for some dinner and then
Some time for a well deserved rest
I've listened to God and done what I can
Selling many books will be the true test

I awake again to the lingering cough
The very one I thought had been gone
But here it is back to remind me once more
Not to push too fast or stretch beyond

My capabilities, which were speeding along
At a pace which I assumed I could handle
But now as I listen to that inner voice speak
I'm quite aware of burning the candle

Its wick is lighting the way for me now
And guiding my feet along the path
I must remember to walk and not run
Or I will certainly run out of gas

And so I am slowing the pace down a bit
I cannot accomplish everything in a few days
Pacing is how every runner wins the race
And I am no different walking through this maize

The pain is lessened, but I am most aware
That every cough tightens up my rib cage
That is where the Fibromyalgia really sets in
And I must remain vigilant to keep it at bay

I take time to pray and to thank our God
For the lessons I'm learning each day
These are true blessings sent directly to me
I simply need to pay attention and pray

Our local newspaper has called this morning
Wanting to do a story about me and "Embracing Life"
I have a long list of contacts to make
I invite them out to learn about pain and strife

The reporter is amazed at my story and how
I have chosen to put into writing in poem
The lessons I've learned throughout the years
Of getting out, moving around and not to bemoan

She seems fascinated that living with three diseases
Has not put me down for too long
Instead I choose to live life to its fullest
As I travel the difficult path towards home

Yes, I have had those long suffering days
Spent entirely flat on my back in bed
But as soon as I'm able, I get going again
I am bound to release these thoughts from my head

And so the writing continues to serve me
And hopefully many others as well
There is always a bright side to every situation
You need just to be open to listen and tell

God is blessing these writings I record
So that others may read and decide for themselves
That no matter how dark it may feel right now
Healing Hope is a state of mind so easily held

I arise very early this morning for me
I will meet with the CEO of our local hospital
I am honored to know him and be his friend
He is the most magnanimous man of all

Leading his team of hospital workers
Always striving to improve how things run
The changes made over the past two years
Are too numerous and prove to be so wonderful

He always makes time to meet with the public
I am so hopeful as I present him with my book
I will meet later with the Cancer Center
For them to give my writings a good look

I'm still moving slowly on this very chilly morn
The temperature is only in the 40's today
Yesterday it was 80 degrees outside
I'm exhausted when I complete the errands on my way

Rest is the calling for the remainder of the day
The coughing has again tired me out
How I long for the day when I can be free
To spend an entire day out and about

Thank you dear God for providing for me
Yet another good day of important meetings
And for reminding me to slow down a bit
So that I may continue my way with warm greetings

"The purpose of life is to believe, to hope, and to strive"
Indira Ghandi

The beginning of the last week in April arrives
I wish the weather was warmer and more sunny
The flowers are just beginning to peek through
And in the garden today, I saw a small bunny

The welcome signs of spring finally appear
Mixed with very wet, chilly and damp days
The leaves are beginning to pop light green
I give thanks to God, with glory and praise

My wheezing remains with me now for weeks
I am amazed at how long a little bug can last
But when one's system is already compromised
Coughing and wheezing can't leave the body too fast

And so I will hope for brighter times ahead
When the garden is finally fully in bloom
The seed catalogues arrive daily in the mail
They always seem to brighten the gloom

It is the time of year to be out of doors
To plant and rake away all the dead leaves
They have served their purpose protecting the plants
When cleared away, they fly in the breeze

Another sign of Healing Hope is here
To see the growth underneath all the debris
The little small flowers are peeping their heads
As if they have at long last all been set free

Yesterday I rested on a bright sunny day
Today it is rainy and unusually chilly
I want to go out and work in the yard
The weather does not cooperate, this is silly

Some energy has returned since I've rested
I tackle cleaning up inside the house instead
The living room is almost back to normal
I am pleased with the progress in my head

I want to always move forward in motion
But lack the ability to judge how high to raise the bar
If I tackle just one small project at a time
I must brake before I've pushed myself too far

This conserving of energy is the right thing to do
But tempering remains a feat for me to overcome
When I start a project, no matter how large
I want it finished before it has even begun

Slow and steady never fail to win the race
We have all read this in old nursery rhymes
Putting those words into practice somehow
Is anything but easy for me during tough times

And so I continue to learn how to manage
To set the right course and the right pace
I continue to pray to God for guidance
And to receive all of His loving good grace

Thank goodness the weather has changed its pattern
A bright sunny warm day has finally arrived
I begin with a trip to the doctor this morning
He is happy to see me looking better and more alive

The next stop is to my former employer
I am greeted by former workers and friends
Many folks choose to purchase my book
A happy surprise for me, I am very content

I am most impressed by a worker and friend
Who has recovered from a very long illness
When last I saw her, she was very near death
It took two entire years for her to achieve wellness

Her weight had dropped dangerously low
She is five foot two inches in height
I believe she had dropped to a mere 76 pounds
And indeed she looked like a total fright

But Healing Hope almost always takes time
She looks so wonderfully bright and alive
I stopped to ask just how much did she weigh
And she proudly said one hundred thirty five

She had to be still, be treated and rest
And wisely she chose to cling to life
God intervened to show her the way
To overcome bitterness and strife

The month of April is nearing its close
It seems to have so quickly flown by
We will all be happy to welcome May
With sunshine and temperatures on the rise

I begin this day with a trip to the hospital
That much needed chest x-ray to finally get
The technician lines me up and says this is easy
Being so thin finally has some real benefit

I return home feeling quite refreshed
The rest of the day is mine to spend however
My brother and I ride out to the nursery
To purchase new rose bushes, each a different color

These will be an early birthday present
For Wilbur, who will celebrate # fifty-seven
Early next week we will go out for dinner
It will be something like being in heaven

He has already chosen the place where we will dine
An Italian restaurant, locally on the Town Green
I must now secretly wrap his other gifts
I know he will enjoy them, they are most serene

I finish the day by raking out the deck gardens
A chore to everyone else but not for me
I so enjoy cleaning up and weeding outside
And looking at the clean beds with glee

The last of April, it is showering and gloomy
A most predictable way for the month to end
For these April showers will bring May flowers
Right around the corner God will surely send

A sign of rebirth, and a chance for us all
To view life from a new perspective
It happens each year, again and again
The chance to begin anew and be selective

This is when New Year's day should be
A true time of renewal and beginning over
When earth springs to life, proving once more
Winter has passed and now there is green clover

My pain level is quite high but so is my spirit
I take time to truly relax, rest and pray
For nothing seems impossible to me right now
I can visualize the next bright sunny day

I believe in miracles and the saying is true
That "All things are possible with God"
His love, His guidance and His blessings abound
Simply get up and slowly look around your yard

I still think of the future that lies ahead
Where Healing and Hope are on top of the list
I imagine taking that meditative walk
Around the labyrinth we plan, what a gift

May Day is here, I wish to string streamers
From the very top of our flag pole
Announcing in many colors to the world
The arrival of Spring has won out over cold

However, it remains damp and dreary today
I read that it will clear up sometime later
I make the most of my time spent inside
Sewing and reading, which is clearly greater

The curtain task is completed and so am I
It is time for a new project and so I forge ahead
I gather some thoughts about the gardens in front
And imagine what they will look like in my head

Remembering our friend Karen who is a gardener
I make a note to phone her early next week
For soon the yard will be ready to accept
A new look and space for flowers to peep

My brother is anxious now that construction is done
To put his wonderful gardening talents to the test
He has the ability to make absolutely anything grow
His love lies in the rare blooming plants the best

The pain is still with me, and yet I carry on
For God is always here right by my side
When I am really in need of a boost, He is still around
Ready to carry me and give me a free ride

A bright sunny morning smiles as I awake
However, it is still exceptionally cool
I have notes to write and letters to send
I begin the day like a full-time working fool

Tonight I will speak at the Athletic Club
A "Motivational Talk" is what it is being called
Because of the exceptionally bad weather we have
I'm duly expecting the talk to be rescheduled

My brother and I head off to run some errands
A stop at the Post Office and then the Bank
Next on the list is the local hardware store
For a Pressure Washer, Wilbur will give thanks

We've already selected the remainder of his gifts
And we hurry home to hide this huge box
In the end, I wrap up the accompanying booklet
And leave the pressure washer in my car trunk locked

As the day progresses, so to does the rain
In fact it is pouring down so fast we need buckets
We arrive at the Athletic Club to find no one there
And we re-schedule my time there for the talk

I must admit to being disappointed at best
This was to be my first speaking engagement
I spent some meaningful time making some notes
They will serve me well in future arrangements

The love of my life celebrates his birthday today
He has chosen to go fishing this morning
He will be accompanied by his good friend Jack
I sense that a deeper relationship is forming

Jack, Roger and my husband Wilbur
Have been friends for over 30 years now
Their friendship has endured the test of time
And I find this truly amazing somehow

Wilbur arrives home from his short fishing trip
And he opens his presents quite joyfully
He looks at the book for the power-washer
And realizes that he now owns one with glee

Later in the day, he gives his new toy a whirl
Testing the power on the worn-out covered deck
He is so impressed with the power of the machine
That he strips the wood down and leaves a mess

Tonight we will treat him to a nice dinner out
He has chosen the place he wishes to dine
I am feeling so blessed from God up above
I sincerely thank Him for this husband of mine

We all have enjoyed our meal out tonight
And I missed not attending aerobics class
What a simple consession for me to have made
To celebrate his birthday with love that truly lasts

"Hope is the thing with feathers, that perches in the soul
And sings the tune without the words and never stops at all"

Emily Dickinson

Hope is a fantastic word for today
Always looking forward with confidence
To trust that your wish will see its way through
To the final joy of fulfillment

Hope is persisting against all odds
That better things are yet in store
We keep it alive in our hearts
For each of us wants nothing more

Although sometimes not easily hope is held
We must constantly learn to strive
Not to focus on pain, whatever it may be
But to trust our spirit and keep hope alive

I am still learning that hope is the way
To live out the rest of my days
I am most thankful for every single moment
That I am alive and able to find new ways

My wish is for all to find and hold onto
The very thing that we call Hope
To treasure its meaning and forever trust
That tested with trials, we will always be able to cope

Today is the fifth day of May
Also known as Cinco de Maya
I am not too familiar with the meaning
But it is celebrated in a remarkable way

Our calendar has always puzzled me so
For the addition of Julius & Augustus Caeser
Were placed so that the remainder of months
No longer correspond with their meanings

September means seven in latin terms
Yet it is the ninth month of the year
October coverts to the number eight
And is the tenth month of the year

November means nine and so it goes
It is the eleventh month of the year
December, which translates to number ten
Is now the twelfth month of the year

Words are intriguing in their own way
I am constantly looking for root meanings
Trivial though it may seem to others
I totally enjoy writing and reading

And so Healing Hope again comes to mind
The word hope in all of its fullness
Lives within me so strongly that
I rest assured in spite of my illness

A most promising day lies ahead for me
A chance at brand new opportunities
To speak with others who suffer with pain
In a complex within a new community

I begin the drive headed almost due north
And end just before reaching the state line
I am meeting with the Activities Director
And find the place to be simply divine

We speak for a while and he loves the book
The message of hope amidst a life of pain
He gives me a detailed tour of the facilities
I definitely want to come and visit again

He is so delighted with my offer to speak
They will set up a book-signing and reception
I'm told there will be 125 people in attendance
We are both mutually pleased beyond expectation

The mere idea of speaking to many different folks
All who suffer from some form of pain
Is a blessing bestowed on me from God above
I look forward to doing this many times again

My ribs are burning, I find myself in pain
I listen to inspirational music on my way
It takes my mind off the pain for awhile
And gives me time to pause, reflect and to pray

A most exciting day has begun
I hope we can each keep up the pace
We are attending a 25th anniversary party
And so off to Manchester begins the race

Our very dear friends Arlene & Fred
Will be renewing their wedding vows
And later they host an elaborate reception ball
Complete with food, music, dancing & flowers

We are seated with some of our closest friends
A chance to finally catch up and converse
And to my delight, many are interested
In my book, which they then offer to purchase

By mid afternoon we head for home
Fifty-three miles to the front door
We all take a short, much needed rest
Before we are again headed out the door

This time we simply walk up the street
To celebrate the birthday of our good neighbor & friend
Bob has reached the grand age of sixty-five
And many number of family and friends will attend

I stay for a long while renewing friendships
While my husband and brother return home
I am enjoying myself and the compliments I receive
I thank God from deep in my very soul

It is Mother's Day and I awake to find presents
From both my dear husband and brother
I receive calls from each of my girls
But I find myself thinking about my mother

I feel her gently smiling down upon us
From heaven where she lives now
She sends down her blessings to each of us
Happy with what she now sees, I humbly bow

She and daddy are delighted to see us
As a family of three taking great care
We are each here to help support one another
I know for certain that they are totally aware

I am also happy to be part of this family
I am blessed from the heavens above
God has graced us and placed us together
We acknowledge the wonderfulness of love

We travel a great distance to spend some time
With Wilbur's mother and sister and others
Mardy & Aunt Ginny, who are both widows
And who immediately fall in love with my brother

God bless all mothers and mothers to be
Their jobs are endless and never, ever done
But blessed we all are to have children to love
Especially grandchildren, each and every one

FOR MOTHER

WHAT IS A MOTHER? SHE IS LOVE
SHE HAS GOD'S BLESSING FROM ABOVE
NO GREATER GIFT COULD HE BESTOW
A CHILD TO LOVE AND HELP TO GROW

UNDERSTANDING, ALL THE WHILE
GUIDING YOU WITH A SMILE
WATCHING YOU GROW, SHE'S ALWAYS THERE
GIVING HER COMFORT AND HER CARE

MENDING HEARTS OR DRYING TEARS
GENTLY HELPING THROUGH THE YEARS
ALWAYS BELIEVING, EVER A FRIEND
A HELPING HAND READY TO LEND

WHAT IS A MOTHER? SHE IS LOVE
SHE HAS GOD'S BLESSING FROM ABOVE
NO GREATER GIFT COULD HE BESTOW
A CHILD TO LOVE AND HELP TO GROW

A start to a new week is finally here
The events of the weekend having been full
Although more hectic than I am used to
I enjoyed myself rather exceptionally well

The fatigue bug has found me, small wonder why
Rest is the mandate for this wonderful day
I would much rather be out spending time in the garden
But must first regain some energy, so I pray

For guidance, compromise, and the patience I need
I lift my heart upwards to hear the words clearly
Now I can simply relax and read for the day
For listen I do, to those words so dearly

I'm learning albeit still slowly to grasp
Each message sent to and from my small body
Knowing what truly is the right thing to do
This day of rest seems like a hot toddy

It serves me well, time to focus and read
The good words that surround me this day
These articles about health, nutrition are sage
They help me to stay on the right path and way

I am finally able to know and discern for myself
What my body needs each and every day
Knowing and adhereing to are two separate things
Thus, I must constantly continue to pray

I awake a sleepyhead, having stayed up too late
Once I start reading, it is difficult to stop
I read quite a long time into the night
And find that I'm certainly not ready to get up

I phone and reschedule the meeting this morning
To next week, much later in the day
I must be fully comprehensible to the client
To grasp what their needs are in a detailed way

I fall back to sleep, though the day is sunny
And do not wake up until almost noon
Now there is a very clear message for me
Sleep deprivation makes me feel like a goon

I find some energy when I finally awake
And busy myself with some ironing and small chores
I realize there are many things on my list
So it is now off to the office supply store

When I return I indulge in a great meal
Consisting of arugula, taboule and turkey
I eat as if this were indeed a gourmet treat
To fuel my body for this evening's work

Class proves a hard workout and I discover
That I must not be fully yet rested
I keep up the pace and sweat like a hog
I am honestly really being tested

Today begins brighter I'm happy to report
I rested quietly after class last night
With ice on my knees, which were sore indeed
To reduce the pain - I looked a bit like a fright

Again I listened and applied the correct treatment
To my knees, overworked and quite distended
I find that by earnestly paying more attention
Healing has become much easier than imagined

The new porch furniture has arrived by truck
The men graciously place it on the back deck
It's just in time as the deck has been cleaned
Power-washed, it is neat and tidy without a speck

Now it is time to head out the door
And pick up my brand new office chair
Why have I waited so long to buy one?
It is truly comfortable beyond compare

My spine is supported along my entire back
And the wheels allow me more freedom of motion
To have been writing in such discomfort before
Ensures that my writing is absolutely my devotion

Thank you dear Lord for this new found comfort
I am sure it will alleviate many a tired night
I'm genuinely quite pleased with myself right now
And am delighted to be able to continue to write

I wake up a little sleepy-head, oh what a gift
Having stayed up late reading again
A surprise when at last I looked at the clock
And found it to be twenty minutes to ten

It is bright, sunny and quite windy outside
Also much cooler for this time of year
I hear that we are expecting a frost tonight
Just when will Spring really appear?

My body senses the weather changing
I do not look forward to the anticipated frost
But I will venture out to class this evening
Hoping to improve my health whatever the cost

Continuity is actually the name of the game
And the persistense to go along with it
The challenge is endless at times it seems
I will not give in to laziness or forfeit

The good works that I have achieved thus far
My weak little muscles beginning to turn strong
My life has new meaning since the writing began
I now know my place and accept where I belong

I continue to thank God for His gifts of grace
That I can see clearly in my every day life
The truth is to count the grace and blessings
Not concentrating on stress, pain, and strife

I did not sleep well during the entire night
And finally get up to write around five
I look at the calendar to find it's Friday the 13th
And the State of Connecticut has lost one more life

Michael Ross, a serial killer, was put to death this morning
His crime was the heinous murder of 8 young women
It gives me pause to think about the death penalty
And the reality that it will not result in crime's end

I am not convinced that an eye for an eye
Is the design for which God intended us to live
Rather, we should pattern our lives after goodness
To love, embrace life, have hope and give

I'm wondering how the victims' families feel now
Does death really bring some closure for them?
The fact that their loved ones are gone from this earth
Is not altered by the lethal injection of this man

I remember reflecting on this very issue
Some fifteen odd years ago now passed
When my friend was attacked by a vicious man
I sat in the courtroom and watched the proceedings aghast

The criminal was sentenced to pay the price
Serving time in a prison for committing this crime
I found that I was filled with disgust and nausea
And needed to exit the courtroom from time to time

God, please have mercy on each of us
As we go about our day to day living
And send down Your kind and loving grace
That we somehow realize life is for loving and giving

(continued on next page)

As I reflect on the state of affairs this day
I am not able to discern what is wrong or right
For death by lethal injection does not seem to match
The heinousness of those never ending nights

When victims were followed, tortured to death
At the hands of a single human being
In our world, good and evil really both do exist
Just what causes a man's mind to swing?

I have an idea of how expensive it actually is
To house, feed and clothe a prisoner for life
Why couldn't the system force these folks to work?
Somehow lessening the burden for you and I

A portion of the funds could be set aside
For victim's aide, recovery and relief
Some victims live the remainder of their lives
In a horrific state of sadness and grief

I find that death seems an easy way out
A paradox, for I am fighting for my life
I must work hard, survival is not easy
I am grateful and happy for each day I'm alive

I will continue to pray for each juror, victim and judge
For each plays a role in the outcome of a trial
And also to pray for the many criminals at large
That justice will win out over the long traveled mile

A beautiful Monday morning has arrived
With sunshine, blue skys and warm weather
It is finally time to work in the yard
We shall do this indeed, all together

I have an early meeting at the Bank
With a past fellow co-worker today
He has promised to help promote my book
I remember to thank God as I pray

When I return home, I change my clothes
To go outside to dig and play in the yard
I find myself unearthing a stone walkway
An archeaological dig, and I didn't travel too far

Since our house was built in the year 1820
The stones were probably placed at the same time
Imagine years of weeds and grass growing
I gain a new perspective of age in my mind

I dig very long before I eventually stop
This play is most labor intensive indeed
I'm glad that I have built up some muscle tone
If not, I would most definitely not succeed

I head straight upstairs to take a shower
And wash off the grime and the dirt
I've managed to accomplish quite a bit
And we are all very pleased with my work

Not usually an early riser am I
But the stones are calling out to me
I continue to dig from eight o'clock till noon
And have reached the end of the walk finally

Once again, I head upstairs to the shower
For I have a meeting scheduled at two
I'm meeting with a woman named Mrs. Love
And a love she proves to be, so very true

We are setting up a date and time to host
A motivational talk and book-signing event
We connect immediately and are on the same page
One and one-half hours time we have spent

I am so delighted to have met this woman
Good new friends we will surely become
Reaching out is the most exciting thing to do
I find it rewarding to meet one on one

She finds my book and the message it brings
To be just what she has been looking for
As the activities director, it is her responsibility
To provide motivation for the seniors she cares for

I think of her along my drive back home
And remember to thank her and to pray
Her job is exhausting to say the least
But she has found a respite this very day

Again, I rise earlier than my usual time
I am scheduled to meet with a wonderful nun
At Wisdom House Retreat and Conference Center
To present her with my book, which is finally done

What a pleasant and inspirational woman she is
With a smile bright enough to light up the sky
We chat for awhile and I visit the chapel
Where I sit very still, praying and asking why

Why have I been blessed with these diseases
Osteoporosis, Osteoarthritis and Fibromyalgia
Yes, I sincerely mean very blessed indeed
My spirit is awakened as I reach out to others

The pain remains with me with each passing day
However, my spirit is becoming very strong
I am no longer distracted by the focus on pain
For I know now exactly where I belong

The Maintenance of my health as best as I'm able
Is my responsibility, which is profoundly loud and clear
With new purpose and focus, I reclaim my life
Looking forward with confidence to each passing year

Thank you dear Lord for allowing me to compose
And be of assistance to others who suffer in pain
Healing hope and prayer are so very powerful
In transforming such acute pain into gain

I awake this morning with enthusiasm and fervor
There are no appointments for me to keep
I choose to go out to the memorial rose garden
To work and weed where the air is ever so sweet

I dig and pull weeds that have become overgrown
Until my arms become too tired to continue
Weeding happens to be my favorite job in the garden
Which is quite a surprise, I imagine, to most of you

It is a cleansing and spiritual process for me
Clearing away the brush, enabling the flowers to grow
By the end of June the gardens will become
A masterpiece from God, to view and to show

My husband and brother are the planters now
With bright sunshine and water and food
It seems to me that a trilogy is formed
We need all three elements to set deep lasting roots

It is not by coincidence that our lives are changed
Around the seasons we each experience new life
How good is our God to allow us this freedom
To constantly improve the quality of our lives

I am moved by the rose bushes so beautiful and lush
With scented flowers and yes, also with thorns
Our lives are likened to the rose bush I believe
We each harbor both secrets and love ever so strong

I'm scheduled to have a full body massage today
I've been looking forward to this day all week
After stretching and straining all my muscles
This will prove to be an extraordinary treat

I bring my own spiritual music to play
And Eileen is ever so delighted to hear it
She begins her work most diligently
And tells me that my body feels fine and fit

She can actually feel definition in those muscles
That I have been working on so hard to rebuild
She tells me that I have a much healthier glow
And I tell her I feel a lot stronger and solid

This is a very relaxing and spiritual hour
That I spend in her exceptionally capable hands
We chat so comfortably with each other
We have, in fact, become very close friends

Wilbur has enjoyed his time in massage
And soon Bert will experience the same
It is the best way I know of to really let go
And totally empty any stress in my brain

I thank the Great Spirit for allowing me this time
It is a prayerful and relaxing hour spent
I am able to feel some healing take place
This is God's gift to me from heaven sent

Wilbur is sick with a sinus infection
He has been put on antibiotics once again
Most of his week was spent traveling
With too much time in the car and the plane

He is finally taking a much needed break
Being forced by the doctor to total rest in bed
This proves to be the best medicine indeed
He sleeps and shuts off everything in his head

How familiar am I with this very concept
Of being forced to lay quiet and sleep
It is usually due to pushing too hard
A promise I have made to myself to keep

I am still learning albeit ever so slowly
To know when to push and when to rest
To not stress my body past its own limits
Remains an ongoing and unrelenting test

Tonight is our monthly trivia game
I drive with Jack & Judy to attend
With only three men and four women playing
The women finally win a game in the end

I arrive home quite late and find Wilbur asleep
I stay up even later, reading and praying
Thanking God for this time spent with friends
Which proved to be ever so entertaining

We are married 11 years and 6 months today
And we are so happy to be with each other
For we are very aware of many past difficulties
Which resulted in us first being brought together

A very dark, cool and damp rainy day it is
But we do not care much about the weather
We are truly grateful for the lives we live
And the fact that we are true partners together

Later this day we will meet with our friends
And will plan for our Celebrate Life Party
Karen and Mark along with my brother
Will share the cost with us to pay for this party

This year will mark the tenth annual event
We look forward to it each and every year
Last year was the first time that we were unable
To host, due to illness, cancer and all of our tears

This year seems so right to celebrate life
Especially for myself, Donna, Judy and Bert
We have each battled some serious health issues
And come out on the other side still alive and pert

Thank you dear Lord for this happy chance
To be able to co-host this great party once again
We have each been blessed with Your loving grace
You have most lovingly reduced our fears and pain

It is colder than yesterday and also quite windy
But, alas it is merely some more of the same
I wonder if I slept through and now it's October
This weather is ridiculous, in fact it's insane

Tonight is aerobics class, I trust that I'll be able
To go and work-out in hopes to get warm
I think we will be doing intervals tonight
Non-stop exercise with weights all evening long

As it turns out that's exactly what we do
It proves to be a regimen hard fought and tiring
I find that my joints don't like this one bit
But I sweat and drink water before retiring

This is the most difficult work-out there is
The moving is continuous with no time to breathe
Finally we relax at the end and do stretching
I'm able to catch my breath by the time we leave

I know this is beneficial for my body's circulation
And building up those weak muscles along the way
I would never push myself this far if working at home
So in the end, I am truly grateful for this day

Again I thank God for this day at its end
When I realize that I've worked very hard
If the sun were shining outside today
I'd have much preferred working in the yard

Today is the day for my complete physical
A slight bit nervous, I take my time getting ready
I simply adore the doctor that I will be seeing
She is thorough, a good listener and rock steady

But I have had too many other issues to deal with
That a complete physical is something I've overlooked
Far too much time has lapsed and gone by
I'd prefer to be reading an interesting book

In fact, that is exactly what I am doing
I bring the book along with me for a distraction
But once I arrive, I share the book with the doctor
She glances through it and says it look fascinating

My blood pressure is taken at 90 over 58
I weigh in at a grand total of 110 pounds
She checks me over completely from head to toe
And then I get to take off my lovely gown

I head straight into her office for the news
Expecting to receive more than one reprimand
But instead she says all signs look good
But she needs to schedule me for a mammogram

She explains that she is not overly concerned
With my weight, I thank God for that
Muscle usually takes much time to build
And eventually will weigh more than fat

MEMORIAL DAY

Today we celebrate Memorial Day
A day to honor all those who have died
Those who have served our country so well
And the many families that have been left behind

I still find it so difficult to truly comprehend
Why we are at war with a nation so far away
One who doesn't value our presence or existence
And our soldiers pay with their lives every day

The lives which have been lost are too many to count
The government will have to erect another Vietnam Wall
To honor those men and women, whose lives have been cut short
In a distant war that seems quite un-necessary at all

"If we have no peace, it is because we have forgotten
that we belong to each other", a quote from Mother Teresa
Have we indeed actually forgotten how to care for
Or to pray for our enemies and each one of us either?

I've been trying to live a more peaceful existence
By putting many names in my little Prayer Jar
Those names of all my friends and also those
I don't care for, and find this most difficult and hard

Bless us dear Lord on this very special day
Lest we forget all those lives which have been lost
And that we face foreign and home enemies too
The price of war never seems to justify the cost

The first day of June and what a delight
A day of reckoning calls to me this morning
I am meeting with a very special group of women
A group I have been searching for and yearning

A bright beginning for a bright new month
This seems such a perfect time of the year
To venture out into territory unknown
To learn about me and perhaps shed a tear

The women are wonderful, listening intently
To everyone who wishes to speak
The reading for the day is lovely and moving
I sit very quietly at place in my seat

But the reading sparks something deep inside
And I find that I'm ready to share
My writing along with my other diseases
Which are at times too much for one to bear

I'm invited to lunch and am delighted to go
We dine at a local breakfast and luncheonette
I'm treated so warmly, we talk and laugh with ease
I am happy to be here at last, comfortable as I can get

I awake quite early this morning to find
Myself very calm and ever so subdued
This is very different from my normal outlook
I ponder the day and feel somewhat amused

There is nothing of major importance
That must be accomplished this day
I head out the door to play in the yard
And six hours later I come in to stay

I have never before enjoyed working outside
The gardening bug has bitten me quite hard
I keep digging and weeding getting ready for
The cedar mulch that I will spread in the yard

I receive a call from a local reporter
Who wants to interview me tomorrow morning
She wants to write a story about me and my book
Which she tells me she finds most charming

I decide that I've worked too much today
And decline to attend my aerobics class tonight
My muscles ache and my back is screaming
I will not push myself over the limit

I phone Cindy to let her know my decision
She is most gracious and tells me to rest
And also not to push myself too hard
For we all know what happens, I fail the test

This morning a reporter came out for a visit
To listen to the story about my first book
She arrived exactly at the allotted time
And she was amazed at how well I look

She was in awe as she looked around the house
And loved the walls of family photos so warm
She found both the house and me to be inviting
She fell in love with the old country charm

My husband came down for part of the talk
Offering his view on Embracing Life and Healing Hope
While this book is mostly about Hopefulness
He said Embracing Life was all about learning to cope

He was himself warm and gracious to our guest
And to me, as is always his way
The reporter said we acted like newlyweds
We truly felt so light, happy and gay

We got back to talking about Embracing Life
She expected to find me crippled in pain
These diseases I have are fortunately invisable
I do battle with every ounce of strength that I can

My story is about accepting changes in your life
Without becoming resentful, bitter and cold
It is certainly directed at making one's self better
Giving yourself permission to live life quite bold

This Saturday morning Wilbur is up at dawn
Getting the car loaded for his annual fishing trip
Together with Roger, Jack and kayaks in tow
The trio drive to a remote spot in Maine, what a hit

It takes a total of ten hours to arrive at their place
They are exhausted from the tedious, long drive
But are most happy to spend this time together
And have been vacationing here since 1975

This is my time to spend however I please
And choose to remain working in the yard
My brother is working right along beside me
As we tackle the tough spots, which are so hard

I find myself up to my elbows in mud and rocks
As I dig out and clear some new places
Everywhere I dig there are rocks to uncover
Dear God, please send me some of Your graces

We take a break to purchase some new plants
We come home and I'm right back to work
I stay digging at this garden until it's suppertime
By that time my entire body is aching and hurt

Thank you God for the energy you have given me
To tackle those huge bags of mulch and chips
I've been hauling them by the wheelbarrow now
To the new gardens one at a time bit by bit

We awake to a very hot muggy day outside
Whatever happened to the time for Spring
The temperature has gone from 50 degrees to 90
There was never a time to allow for this swing

So of course it feels like the middle of summer
With the humidity high it causes us to sweat
Nonetheless, we continue our work outside
Since there remains so much work to be done yet

I find that I'm drinking gallons of water
To replenish the amout that I am losing
I layer on the bug spray and head out the door
After coming in for a very short dozing

I am careful to not work in the middle of the day
The heat then is too hot and strong to bear
I have gained a new perspective for all those folks
Who work outside all day year after year

I thought that growing up in south Florida
Would acclimate me to the summers up north
But I forget that we reside so far inland
There are no ocean breezes to cool us off

Thank you again God for just one more day
To play in our gardens, which are becoming
Many places to enjoy all that You have given
To wander through each day lazily by roaming

This day marks the beginning of a very important week
Karen, my friend the gardener, is escorting me to
The wholesale place where she purchases for her clients
She has drawn a plan, but there are so many things to look through

Finally we decide on some Dwarf Alberta Spruces
Along with some Azaleas and Hydrangeas
Then we select a Chamacyperous Tree
And some Holly bushes and Rhododendrons

These will be placed all along the front yard
Near the house and along the new addition
These places have been barren for 186 years
And now the front yard will look like heaven

I am fortunate as Karen passes on her discount to me
We would never be able to pay the full retail price
I am thankful for her friendship and all that it means
Good friends are God's blessings within our lives

We come home and unload all the purchased bushes
And put them in their respective new places
Now comes the time for digging and planting
That will have to wait for another few days

For shortly a photographer is coming out
To take a few pictures of me for the news
The reporter has already written her article
Now they need a good photo, I am amused

I peek out this morning to see if the plants are still there
And low and behold to my total surprise
I find that the racoons have toppled all the garbage
And I must rake the mess up before the trash men arrive

I quickly put on my heavy garden gloves
And find a rake strong enough to handle this mess
I gag as I go about raking up the trash into the cans
I've never before been put to this kind of test

I head back inside, the mess finally cleaned up
And find I have no appetite for breakfast
I sit for awhile and sip on some coffee
It will be some time before I'm hungry at last

Back to the gardens I head for the day
As one job is completed, I seem to create another
This could turn out to be bigger than I thought
Thank God for the assistance of my brother

We work quite well together at this thing
His gardening knowledge far surpasses mine
And so I always ask before continuing on
Where should we plant this flower or vine?

He is always there to offer his guidance
Which I readily accept as the garden gospel
He has been at this for many more years than me
I'm still a novice at this as anyone can tell

Today I'll attend my women's support group meeting
We meet every Wednesday morning at eleven
The group is smaller than usual this bright sunny day
Some women are away on vacation or travel

My pain and fear are diminishing quickly
As I look forward with much greater hope
Healing takes time, I have come to accept
I'm on my own journey and have been set afloat

I stop at the Agway on the way home
To pick up more bags of cedar mulch and pine chips
I've begun the task of weeding out the walkways
In the vegetable garden between the beds lifted

I will first lay down some gardening cloth
And then spread a deep layer of small pine chips
This should hopefully keep the weeds at bay
And I'll have more time to work on the Labyrinth

A Labyrinth is something that I've always wanted
And now that some large bushes have been dug up
There is plenty of room for this meditative walk
I simply have to set the plans on paper with chalk

The gardens are finally beginning to show
The hard work, which so far has been done
I long for the time when we can sit and relax
And truly admire and enjoy our time in the sun

I can hardly wait to have breakfast and go outside
Although it is a sweltering 90 degrees
I do not mind, as I want to dig and plant
Another day to spend in the garden as I please

I've been working very hard alongside my brother
While Wilbur is away on his fishing trip
Trying to get so very many things done
But realizing at what time we must quit

I find that I must bow to my body's limitations
To not overdo is most difficult for me
My mind tells me to continue right along
While my body speaks entirely differently

The mind and body must work hand in hand
In order to not become completely fatigued
Why oh why is this lesson so hard to grasp?
Dear God please answer this question for me

I can feel Your presence as I plod along
With the weeding and laying down the mulch
Your voice of encouragement helps to motivate me
While Your words of wisdom tend to make me gulp

I know that I must adhere to Your words
Please help me as I attempt to really listen
I treasure my faith and do place my trust in it
The gardens are beginning to glisten

Today I will meet with my good friend and counselor
Who has assisted in my growth pattern to date
While never telling me exactly what to do
She leaves me to discover my own fate

I am so comfortable with her I hold nothing back
And our discussions are honest and true
She helps me to see another perspective of life
And in so doing, helps to widen my point of view

There is always another way to see one's life
If one takes the time to seek and find
Everything we need to improve ourselves
Is waiting, if we do not remain blind

Growing in faith, love and hope each new day
Has become my mode of accepting who I am
No longer worrying about the things I cannot do
But being grateful for the things that I can

Life has become a wonderful place
I look forward with much greater hope
To be contented with what I have in life
And possess the tools which help me to cope

Thank you dear Lord for giving me this time
To re-evaluate my life along this new pathway
To continue to discover and grow deep inside
Is Your blessing to me each and every day

The weekend is upon us once again
The time to relax and enjoy as we please
I am working so very diligently again
I'm loving the outdoor flowers and trees

When Wilbur returns home later this evening
I know that he will be simply amazed
At all the work which has been accomplished
He will walk around the gardens in a daze

He does not disappoint me at all on this
As he walks through an entire week's work
He cannot believe what he sees with his eyes
And asks me "who moved all the dirt"?

I tell him that Bert and I worked together
He hesitates as he looks around again
Knowing that neither of us has the strength
And then asks me if I'm in very much pain?

I tell him that it was a work of love
God provided the muscle that I needed
He is grateful for what he no longer must do
And still cannot believe how much land was weeded

He had a great time on his fishing vacation
And Bert and I had a wonderful week as well
There remains a lot of work still ahead to be done
I find myself singing "The Farmer in the Dell"

Another bright and sunny day is upon us
The temperature is in the 90's once more
We have now had more hot days during this time
Than there were all of last summer before

Wilbur gets up and makes pancakes for breakfast
A real treat since we've not bothered to cook
We all sit down at the table together
To devour our breakfast and thank the cook

Wilbur walks outside to view the gardens
In utter amazement, he shakes his head
He cannot conceive of the work that's been done
And looks twice more to observe the well tended beds

I am delighted to see him this happy
It's amazing that a true labor of love
Can bring such satisfaction to me
A blessing from the Great Spirit above

Now it is his turn to accomplish some chores
He continues to look all around the yard
I tell him just how many bags of mulch we bought
Which have all been used in our working so hard

He volunteers to go to the garden supply store
To purchase 12 more bags of mulch of rich red cedar
I tell him that those will be used in one day's time
He realizes at once how much more will be needed

The beginning of a new week is here
A chance to embrace opportunity once again
Although my body has been working very hard
I allow myself no time to focus on the pain

Rather, I am grateful for this brand new day
To seize my life however it may appear
I no longer focus on what I cannot do
Rather on what I can do that has become so dear

As I look around me I finally realize
Just how abundantly blessed I have become
To find such pleasure in life's smallest things
I know for certain that my battle has been won

The illnesses that I live with I now consider small
In comparison to my strong will to succeed
I refuse any longer to live in such great fear
God has graced me with many blessings indeed

The blessings of hope and faith remain strong
And I must share my story with many others
Those who are bitter about pain and who stay
Locked in fear trembling under the covers

There is so much of life surrounding us each day
If we are only but grounded in trust and love
We must wake ourselves up to see the real beauty
That life is for living, a message sent from heaven above

It is Flag Day today in our United States
Thankfully I can see many flags flying
I pause to reflect on the war in Iraq
And remember all those who are dying

The media is filled with such dreadful reports
I scan the paper for some glimpse of good news
I find it most difficult to read the paper
The stories of good deeds remain few

Do Americans really need to read and to view
The horror in the nation and the world?
How about the stories of everyday heroes
Let's hear about them while our flag is unfurled

The world today is a very different place
Than the one I grew up with as a child
It is filled with hate, murder and mayhem
Where are those citizens, meek, humble and mild?

We should be taking every opportunity known
To acknowledge the good works of so many
Those stories seldom make the front page
I would gladly pay to hear good news, if any

I will bow my head in prayer this very day
And pray that this ridiculous war is soon over
We are so focused on winning we forget
The olive branch of peace is in our power

The day for my dreaded mammogram has arrived
It's been too many years since the last one I had
I know it is very important to my overall health
I feel irresponsible and somehow very sad

With two friends now recovering from breast cancer
I tell myself that this test will be quick and easy
My other health issues have taken a front seat
How is it I have taken life so carefree and breezy?

The testing is done and I await the results
My body forms tumors and cysts like fingernails
It plays a game called "let's find a new spot"
My strength and faith in God must prevail

Thankfully, everything is "normal" I'm told
I am so grateful I break down in tears
I feel guilty having neglected this part of my health
For far too long and too many years

Another disaster I have fortunately escaped
Thank you God for sparing me this scare
You now have my full attention once more
To be mindful of my body and to be aware

I have learned quite a lot over the past two years
About accepting things which cannot be changed
I'm reminded each day of the Serenity Prayer
And remain hopeful for the things I am able to change

Another lovely day has been given to us
I'm going to have my hair colored and cut
A visit to Doug is always such great fun
He is loving and funny, a real coconut

He has saved the news article about me and my book
Of course, his name is mentioned in it as I tell
He jokes and tells me when I talk about him
I should always reveal the name of "Headlines" as well

We laugh and joke in our usual manner
As he cuts my overgrown mop of hair
It has become so thick, it needs to be thinned
As my mom used to say, thick head – thick hair

I bring him some birthday balloons and a card
No one in the shop has remembered at all
His 35th birthday is really tomorrow
He is thankful for my cheerful gift and call

He talks about his upcoming wedding
To Carissa, the love of his life
He can hardly wait until September
When she will become his lovely wife

I find myself very excited for both of them
He describes the place where they will marry
I'm familiar with the hall and know very well
That it will be a beautiful event, not to worry

The week is drawing to a close today
Tomorrow begins the long awaited weekend
The heat and humidity have not broken in days
We really need a break in the weather to bend

These long, hot days have become overbearing
It is difficult to work so hard out of doors
But we continue on with a slower pace
There remain so many uncompleted chores

Our "Celebrate Life" party is one month away
The property has become completely renewed
People stop by to comment on the beauty
And I take in the splendor of the new views

We have each worked so hard during this month
I am often left very tired and weak
But flowers now bloom in parts of the yard
Which before looked so barren and bleak

Wilbur is amazed each time he walks out
To see what has been accomplished in a day
When he returns home from a business trip
He is so often totally blown away

He knows my strengths and my limits too
And realizes that I have been pushing hard
He reminds me gently to take a break
I look up at him, giving a friendly smile and nod

It is trivia game night at Alice and Bob's
I begin baking the much loved lemon cake
We all bring something to contribute to dinner
I am the appointed one usually asked to bake

I get this done in the early morning hours
As I know that the day will be quite humid and hot
Now I am free to go "play" in the yard
I can return outside to the unfinished spot

My hands are stiff and the joints are locked
I must ice them down before I can start
I take out my bags of peas from the freezer
And place one underneath, the other on top

This helps to reduce the inflamation at once
But I am aware and heed to the warning
I put on garden gloves and go outside
I adhere to my limits, careful to avoid harming

My knees take the brunt of the work today
As I am protecting my hands from the work
It is both fun and yet tiresome for me
To go outside and play in the dirt

Thank you dear Lord for the time to come in
Get showered and rest up for a bit
The trivia game goes head to head
But the women finally win, what a hit

Oh blessed Sunday, to sleep in late
No schedule to follow, simply relax and rest
To browse through the papers and read the news
While looking through sales flyers, who has the best?

I spend a very lazy morning sipping good coffee
And then I devour some really great toast
This is the best part of the day, which I savor
It's a peaceful morning, the kind I love the most

It is a sunny, bright, and unusually warm day
I am delighted to remain inside and read
Although there are a million chores to complete
Nothing is calling me to respond to a need

I breathe in the clean air wafting through the door
And can even smell the rugusa roses, so sweet
What a gift from God to experience this day
It is a most exceptionally unexpected treat

I choose only to read the good news I can find
And pass up the horrible news of the war
It's not that I don't want to be uninformed
I am seeking stories to brighten my very core

Thank you God for the comic strips today
Although they are often politically driven
They provide some humor in this scary world
I long to see families who are loving and giving

The beginning of a very busy week is here
One filled with book promotions and talks
I am greatly looking forward to this work
I have experience and can easily walk the walk

God has provided me with another opportunity
To reach out to many other folks in need
To stand up in front of a fairly large crowd
And to share my personal vision of hope indeed

I am relaxed at the thought of speaking again
Having previously done so in my former line of work
But it was something required of me then
This time it is my own choice to help those who hurt

I gather my materials together to prepare
I don't want to be scurrying around last minute
Once I have everything collected together
I am free to put my mind at rest and begin

I spend the rest of the day in the gardens
Working at my own slow pace
Little by little the work will get done
I have learned that there is no great race

I am finished for the day and come inside
Take a warm shower and wash my hair
I am smitten at once by the falling water
And God's soft and refreshing clean air

I arise fairly early to begin this day
And choose to spend time in the yard
I must come back in by eleven thirty
For my first talk, hopefully it won't be hard

My husband is accompanying me to the place
Where I will give my motivational speech
He asks if I know what I'm going to say
I answer "I'll know by the crowd I'm going to reach"

He is an excellent presenter himself
This is part of his work and profession
Always having a planned program on which to rely
He is interested to hear how I'll do once I'm on

The elderly people file in one at a time
Some using walkers and others just smiling
I walk around the room greeting some folks
I now know what it is I'll be saying

I am graciously introduced by the director
And begin to address the crowd right away
I welcome them and give them a glimpse of cheer
This is one bright and brilliant day

I begin by asking their definition of pain
And then move quickly to the subject of hope
I tell them about my book "Embracing Life"
That it tells the story of learning to cope

I awake groggy from a long night's sleep
And am grateful for the opportunities this day
I will take my brother to see the specialist
For his evaluation and to listen to what he has to say

Later this evening I will have the chance
To speak with some seniors about my book
I love the opportunity to talk about hope
To meet the audience and capture them with a hook

I tell them that if I were simply to ask
Their definition of what pain is to them
That I would likely hear as many different answers
As there are people in attendance, Amen

I reinforce that pain takes on many faces
Physical, emotional and different folks
There are as many different kinds of pain
As there are musical keys and piano notes

And so I focus on healing our outlooks on life
To count our blessings to be alive this day
To find the love and hope within ourselves
Always proves to be the correct thing, I say

They listen intently as I move from the podium
To circulate amongst the good people here
Most of them are smiling back at me
It feels so natural to be standing right here

It is Friday, a beautiful bright, sunny day
I'm still thinking about last night's engagement
A delightful reception was held in my honor
After my short talk and book-signing event

I remember to thank the Activities Director
Via special e-mail sent directly to Scott Zbell
The entire evening was a most pleasant adventure
It was planned and executed quite well

I choose to spend some time in the gardens
They are all just growing in God's great light
With a mix of rain, sunshine and tender care
And new solar panels to light them at night

I remain in awe of the beautiful flowers
And now believe that cultivating the soil
Is akin to cultivating one's soul as well
The result is worth every bit of effort and toil

God has clearly shown His face to me
And with it a new opportunity for hope
I believe with every tiny cell of my body
That there is no greater gift than Hope

The weekend is upon us once again
Wilbur has arrived home safe and sound
I always pray harder each time he travels
That he will return and land safely on the ground

He has many chores that he is working on
Thus he rises early and is out to the barn
For that is where his wood-working shop is
He works diligently, safe and protected from harm

He is making some new built-ins for brother Bert
And his work is all dedicated with love
He is grateful to have Bert here with us
Surely this is God's grace to us from above

I can feel the sense of brotherly love
Getting stronger with each passing day
What a gift and blessing we all have here
I remember to thank God and continue to pray

For my brother's health seems to be improving
I think gardening is so very good for his being
His knowledge of plants is overwhelming to me
He knows what will grow where without first seeing

Thank you dear Lord for my husband and brother
And for the gifts You continue to bestow on us
Everything seems to simply fall into place
With Your grace, there is little trouble or fuss

Sunday is here, I'm reminded of a day to rest
Surely we must take advantage of the good weather
My brother and I choose to tend the gardens with delight
My husband is at work building a new cedar chest

It will also become a new window seat for Bert
Underneath the short window between his closets
Or perhaps it will be a seat for his cat "Miss Mary"
To take her sunbath and look outside at the flowers

In any event, Wilbur is utilizing every tiny bit of space
To ensure that every square inch has been efficiently used
What a wonder to see just how he accomplishes this feat
The built-ins are in place and each built for a specific use

He comes over to check on our gardening chores
And is totally amazed at what has been done so far
He cannot imagine that I have lifted and carried
The bags of mulch, but I have since raised the bar

I bend with my legs and lift that way also
Being very careful to not strain my back
Bending and lifting I learned in aerobic's class
I move forward with strength that I previously lacked

I thank our dear Lord for another good day
I stop working before I am completely spent
A nice cool shower brightens my spirit
I am grateful for this time, which is heaven sent

A brand new day, a brand new week
I wonder what treasures are in store?
God has led me safely thus far
But I seem to want so much more

More time to play in the sun again
To continue my work in the yard
I am praying that my energy level
Will allow me to press on and go far

I have now learned the lesson so hard to embrace
Of when to work and when to stop for a break
This digging and planting and spreading mulch
Is by no means simply a "piece of cake"

It is very hard work, but I am able to find
Such reward in the beauty that will last
For by planting so many perennial plants
They will return again, with even more flash

The first year they bloom with modesty
While taking time to set their roots
When spring-time comes again next year
They will have begun to send out new shoots

God is clearly watching over me
By sending His blessings and love
I am humbled by the grace that He has sent
From His magnificant home up above

Another bright day, we are fortunate indeed
Last summer proved to be quite damp and cold
Although these days are hot and humid
This is what summer is all about we are told

I remember my youth spent in south Florida
With humidity almost unbearable to take
But here in the northwest hills of Connecticut
We can always cool off with a swim in the lake

This is clearly the most exquisite place to live
To experience the thrill of four seasons
I never really appreciated Spring before
But find every day, many new reasons

Summer began less than one week ago
And many are complaining of all the heat
I remember the cold and wet Spring we had
This to me is a time to rejoice and greet

I am amazed at the accomplishments we have made
To enhance our property with such great beauty
The addition itself has prompted improvements
With wonderful space for much fun and utility

May God continue to bless us all
As our work is a dedication of love
To have my brother living here with us
In his own space, graced from above

I awake and gaze out at the Memorial Rose Garden
And remind Wilbur to clean up the name plates
For every rose has been planted for someone
No longer with us, but passed on through the gates

Out in front is the rose bush for all our kitty friends
With "Ferris", the iron cat standing guard in place
The remainder of the bushes are a constant reminder
Of those we love, we can clearly see each smiling face

There are family, friends and neighbors too
Each rose having its own special name plate
Our neighbor has three family members here
Three too many for one family to take

Wilbur's dad and my dad are behind one another
I am struck by the smell of cigars and pipes
Each time I pass by their beautiful rose bushes
I feel their presence, as if they were alive

My mother's rose bush is a gorgeous bright color
She never wore anything dark, drab or dull
I can easily feel her smiling down on us
Her roses are a delightful shade of vibrant coral

Two new bushes were added just this year
One for Anthony and one for "Uncle Don"
I can hardly wait until their family members
See remembrances of their loved ones now gone

Today I am scheduled for a full body massage
I can barely wait until two o'clock
Wilbur is also having a massage this day
His is scheduled for eleven o'clock

I am headed off this morning to my women's group
We meet each Wednesday morning at the church hall
The reading this morning is about "self pity"
I am anxious and ready to share with all

I find self pity to be an absolute waste of time
Why not focus on our accomplishments instead?
For although we have all asked the question "why me"
We'd be better off praying and bowing our heads

I know that whenever I host a pity party
I'm the only one who is in attendance
Wouldn't it be better to host a real party?
Where we could all gather to sing and dance

I speak up and say what is on my mind
And notice others nodding in agreement
Everyone surely has achieved something small
To be grateful for with time well spent

I thank God for all my blessings to date
Counting my accomplishments and failures too
All these things have led me to where I am
I know there is much more that I can do

I can hardly believe that so much of the year has passed
Much has happened, the time has simply flown by
When I look back to the initial day of January first
The changes we have encountered seem to pile up high

We have dealt with death, illness, and love
Each of us holding the other up somehow
I do a mental count of events, month by month
And find it difficult to believe where we are now

God truly has a plan set for each one of us
However, we are unaware of just what that plan is
We simply accept life one day at a time
Remembering that we are here to love and to give

Our days string along, most with great purpose
Along with those days we are instructed to rest
I find that I pay more attention to each day now
Finding life is for living, and is not a constant test

As each day passes there are opportunities for us
Decisions to make that will affect our lives
We do the very best in our decision making
Asking for wisdom from the Great Spirit, our Guide

I am grateful and happy just to be me
Free to accomplish or fail at whatever I take on
I am certain that God will forgive my mistakes
As long as I strive to be the best person I can

Today is the day I've been long waiting for
I will spend most of the day at the bank
The folks are hosting a book-signing open house
With a reception, what a pleasant event

I shower and dress with the utmost care
Selecting a pretty yellow flowered dress
I have boxes of books to take along with me
Hoping to sell many, as the day progresses

The day passes slowly, but I manage to meet
A few interesting people along with the bank president
In the end, I sell only a mere seven books
But have been given the entire day in which to rest

I have made some very important connections
While the press is there taking our pictures
I met a man who runs his company for his employees
And find he is in the same line of work, giving lectures

And then a lovely woman appeared to me
She had read about the book signing affair
She found it hard to believe it wasn't being held
At the local bookstore, which is no longer there

Thank you again God for this chance to meet
With people who suffer with daily pain
I am certain that my book along with kind words
Will provide encouragement for all to try again

The beginning of another celebration weekend
It looks to be sunny and bright all the way through
Hopefully, everyone will keep safety high on the list
The police force will be out and about with their full crew

I will take time this day to spread chips and mulch
Being very careful to not over extend myself
For tomorrow my friend and her children will come
I am working very hard, like a little Santa Elf

I want the yard to look beautiful and thus
Am doing some finishing touches all around
I can no longer keep track of the total number of bags
Of cedar mulch and pine chips spread on the ground

Today I am working under the two lilac trees
Having cleared a large space underneath
Planting perennials and rocks in their proper places
Spreading cedar mulch to make everything look neat

The front yard now looks like a work of art
With plantings all along the front of our home
And gardens alongside of the stone walkway
Now a garden with lilac trees to cover like a dome

Thank you God for the opportunity to improve our home
A little old farmhouse set far back out of the main town
Where we see all forms of wildlife appear
Deer, racoon, bear, and birds, who sing their lovely song

A Celebration Day?

Our troops are fighting and loosing their lives
There is so much work to be done here at home
I wonder why we are involved in this war at all
What kind of world has this truly become?

When men and women are giving up their lives
In a country that doesn't seem to want our aide at all
American's are spit at in disgust in these places
Many will not return home to see the beautiful Fall

Our President is loosing faith with our people
He seems to have an agenda all his very own
It is difficult to view the scenes of terror on the news
I think it is time for our troops to return home

I honestly pray daily for peace all over the globe
Wars have been going on since the beginning of time
Why is it that we are involved in these power struggles?
Have we all become so apathetic and blind?

Many parades are held all over the country today
Celebrating our independence and our win
For freedom of rights and equality for all
Just when will this freedom and equality begin?

The Friday of another weekend begins
It is one week until our big "Celebrate Life" party
We continue our work in the yard and gardens
It is back-breaking work, but we are all hearty

Hearty in mind at least, if no other place
The bags of pine chips are extremely heavy
I call upon my deceased father for his wisdom
His advise comes at once and I am now ready

He tells me to tip the wheel-barrow on its side
And roll the pine bark chips into the wheel-barrow
Now all that is left is to push the entire load upright
It works, I smile up at the sky with my eyes narrowed

I expect to see his face smiling down at me
For I seldom listened when he was alive
He taught me to think and live quite independently
And now I seek his wisdom and sage advise

The rest of the day is tiring and long indeed
But I have overcome what I thought was impossible
One merely needs to learn to ask for help
And everything soon becomes possible

Today I am called outdoors once again
The air is breezy but very humid and warm
I remain amazed at my longing for the sun
And protect myself from the ray's harm

To plant a garden and watch it grow
Is a beautiful act of true hope
The flowers are now in exquisite bloom
I see God's wonder wherever I look

My brother has had a great deal of pain
But his hope lies in the flowers he plants
He looks forward to each and every morning
When he steps out on his deck and stands

He looks like the king of a manor somehow
Overlooking the yard with great pride
I know that it brings him healing and hope
And makes him feel better inside

We are grateful for this time we spend together
Working side by side, sister and brother
We laugh and play as little children do
Our love for each other is evident to others

The days draw nearer for our "Celebrate Life" party
There remain many last minute things to be done
We're trying to accomplish them early in the week
So that we are rested when the day finally comes

We plod along doing what we can each day
And are tired and quite sore at day's end
We will get up tomorrow and try again
All the while learning how to give and bend

It has rained and the bags of mulch are heavy
I resort to my father's great wisdom
But I find that laying down the black weed cloth
Pushes my limits, I finally adhere to them

Talk about bending, I feel like "Gumby"
Bending and stretching for all I'm worth
But slow and steady and taking some breaks
Give me confidence to continue with my work

Planting flower gardens is fairly easy work
Tending the surrounding grounds is hard
Weeding is absolutely grueling for me
But something so rewarding, I thank God

For the ability to stay with the task at hand
And to pace myself and drink in much water
To prevent the chance of any dehydration
And to gaze out in total wonder and awe!

The day to Celebrate Life is upon us
We should all be celebrating life daily
The band arrives to begin their set-up
Yes, now I believe even more fervently

The woman we hire to take care of the kitchen
Arrives with her beautiful smile and good cheer
How fortunate we are to put on this event
Where everyone eats plenty, drinks soda or beer

I look out on the yard and find people everywhere
Some play horseshoes and some play badminton
There are those who are dancing on the deck
And those content to sit and simply listen

The music rings out over the entire place
The gardens are stunningly beautiful
There is more food than all can consume
We are blessed to have friends and food so plentiful

We greet each guest and spend time with them
They are all quite special to us indeed
There were between 75 – 100 family and friends
Enjoying the day, we were most pleased

Before retiring completely for the night
I thank God for this most blessed day
A sense of peace and tranquility flows within
I am ever grateful, I smile as I pray

Ninety Three years old is Grandma today
Very bright and sharp as a tack she is still
She cannot believe she has lived this long
We, as family are all more than thrilled

We travel for brunch being held for a friend
As she celebrates her 60th birthday
Linda is totally surprised as she arrives
Everyone had sealed lips with nothing to say

The brunch was hosted by her beau and daughter
Which proved to be quite a lovely affair
A grand old time was had by everyone
We totally enjoyed the company we shared

We are tired out when we finally return home
In part due to the party held yesterday
How blessed we are to have 2 celebrations
We are thankful and remember to pray

Thank you dear God for family and friends
For reasons to celebrate life so well
We phone dear Granny to wish her greetings
She too has enjoyed her day as well

How wonderful to have previously scheduled
A total hot oil body massage for this day
My body is suffering from the recent events
It is with true thanksgiving that I happily drive away

I arrive at the therapist's a few minutes early
She greets me with her good natured smile
And tells me again just how much she enjoyed
Our "Celebrate Life" party, which was a ball

I am so ready to have her knead out the soreness
Which has resided in my body for weeks
The yard-work has indeed taken its toll
I lie down, relax and am unable to speak

She begins with her healing hands on my back
And feels the bubbles popping at once
These are nitrogen bubbles filled with poison
I can feel her healing hands working out the knots

She works so diligently over my body
Finding more tightness than I was aware
I am grateful and want to stay much longer
I remember to thank Eileen in my prayers

"Happiness is the meaning and the purpose of life,
The whole aim and end of human existence"
Aristotle

Amongst the tears of sorrow and joy
True happiness exists for each and all
By training our minds to look for the good
We avoid the temptation to fall

Gloom and a state of total despair
Are not the places that God intended
Trying to keep a smile on one's face
Even if it is one that's pretended

The news is full of horror enough
With articles, which are so very glum
Try to pick up an inspirational story
See what your new viewpoint will become

I would much rather read a tale with meaning
Than the front page news in the paper
The best stories are most often hidden
In the midst of or near the back of said paper

When all else fails, I read about miracles
For I do believe they validly exist
For when I find them, my mind is changed
And so are the things on my "to do" list

"All time spent angry is time lost being happy"
Mexican proverb

Continuing on the theme of happiness
Is so cleansing for everyone's soul
To focus anew with fresh hope in hand
Looking forward to learn what will unfold

We are each responsible for our own happiness
No matter the many troubles that may befall
If life did not deal us any difficulties
We would never appreciate the good at all

It is simply a matter of balance in our lives
Treading along that treacherous balance beam
It seems so easy for us to get knocked off
And forget our most precious dreams

God calls us to live the best that we can
With happy and fulfilling lives to lead
Of course there are times of hurt and doubt
To emulate the good, is to succeed

No matter one's faith or lack thereof
We should expect for happiness to rule
With an open mind towards our fellow man
Is to feed ourselves the necessary fuel

"Our chief want is someone who will inspire us
to be what we know we could be"
Ralph Waldo Emerson

Emerson issues a challenge with his words
Who is it that inspires you and me?
Reading his many works of wisdom
May somehow set each of us free

Find those people, who influence your life
And pay little heed to those who complain
For they seem to take the very joy of life
And wash it all away down the drain

To surround one's self with wisdom and hope
Is the greatest way to boost how you are feeling
But listening is the most important thing of all
To absorb those wise words, which often bring healing

To dwell in possibility has become my mantra
Constantly looking forward with hope
No matter what blows life has in store
I am confident that I will be able to cope

I thank God for His healing and Hope
For all the blessings He has bestowed
To be secure and hold on to my faith
Positively helps in lightening the load

"In Summer, The Song Sings Itself"
William Carlos Williams

We are one month into the season of summer
And true summer weather is here at last
Flower gardens are in magnificant bloom
The birds sing as we hold onto life fast

Heat and humidity honestly feel fabulous to me
Many signs appear, that we might appreciate life so well
Because Spring passed us by this year
The lush green of summer whispers softly to tell

That God is present in everything that we see
Green lawns, green trees, and the many fragrant blooms
I've never fully appreciated the summer season before
Many are complaining of the hazy days that loom

Rebirth is clearly the message God is sending
We are able to be reborn in this glorious season
And look at life through clear sightned eyes
A chance to think anew with wisdom and reason

I am humbled by the vistas I now can see
From the passage of long bitter cold winter days
To feel God's warmth and serenity surround me
I kneel in thanksgiving, offering my humble praise

"No matter under what circumstances you leave it, home does not cease to be home. No matter how you lived there-well or poorly"
Joseph Brodsky

I am looking at home in a brand new way
A harbor of safety, warmth and love
Truly knowing the people with whom I reside
Are God's gifts and blessings sent from above

It is an honor to have loving family and friends
To love, cherish and to live with each day
I am cognizant of the blessings they provide
And remember at day's end to thank God and pray

We are happy together, the three of us
In our old farmhouse made of chestnut beams
We share the chores and fun almost equally
There is no better life that we could possibly dream

God has renewed each of us in His time and place
We acknowledge His work as we pray
We each have been given the graces we need
To live freely in each endeavor along the way

Counting each blessing is easily done
Not forgetting the pain along the way
I count those times as blessings too
They teach me how sincerely I must pray

"It is only when you start a garden that you realize that
something important happens everyday"
Geoffrey B. Charlesworth

I've spent many days now thinking of gardens
And yes, the truth above must be told
To tend very carefully, watching in time
As each tiny bud begins to unfold

Something great really does happen
Beneath the ground and within our hearts
Tending to each plant begging each to bloom
And treating each other as plants from the start

It's amazing to me how when we care for a garden
Our relationships with others become more tender
We become softer and kinder with those we meet
We share more openly, God has chosen us the sender

The sender of His love and marvelous work
With those who take the time to share
We could not possibly grow a garden of love
Without sunshine, rain and tender care

Thank God for gardens and the lessons they teach
That every single day is important in some way
We come to appreciate so very much more
And as day ends, we remember to pray

"Neither a lofty degree of intelligence nor imagination nor both together are the meaning of genius. Love, love, love, that is the soul of genius"
Wolfgang Amadeus Mozart

Ah, to know that the soul of love is genius
Love, flowers, and music are so true
Gifts given freely to each one of us
Vibrant colors in many a beautiful hue

We need merely to open our hearts to receive
In our souls, the wonderful gift of love
And to share that love with every one
This is truly a blessing from above

Imagine the love of the great composers
Whose creative music stirs us to life
With great vision we are able to truly see
The love in their souls along with their strife

This is exactly the point that we all share
Great moments and sad times together
We are not exempt from the happenings
Of moments which bring changes like the weather

We are called to love, the course of mankind
To both accept it and also to share
How wonderful is this thing called "Love"
To lose it, I could not bear

Happy Birthday Daddy in Heaven

I'm remembering my wonderful dad today
He would have been one hundred and three
A great and wise man he was on this earth
Teaching me how to really live free

Of the many lessons he taught to me
I believe that the greatest one of all
Was to think and act independently
And to reason out any difficulty or fall

Daddy was a very thin and tall man
And his carriage was most impressive
It did not matter what clothes you wore
Rather it was love that made you a success

His heart was pure as were his words
A man of integrity he certainly was
He spoke honestly and truthfully
He believed in purpose and cause

He lives with me still as I hear his words
When I ask for his assistance with a problem
He chides me a bit, telling me to reason it out
And eventually come to the right solution

As I gaze up at the stars late at night
Each constellation he points out to me
Naming them each one after the other
If I look very carefully, I am able to see!

Welcome Baby Eve

A brand new baby Eve has just arrived
Another precious life has begun
Her arrival has touched many already
And so bursts forth the many years of fun

This special ocassion for which we have waited
Is a most pleasant surprise for us all
Eve arrived a week and one-half late
We anticipate the future having a ball

The fairest of skin and a mop of hair
Are the very first pictures we have seen
Another gift sent from heaven above
Her parent's eyes filled with pride do beam

Wilbur will see her sometime next week
I can barely wait to hold her myself
This child is his very first grandchild
She reminds me of a tiny little elf

She is perfect and healthy, a blessing indeed
Such joy does this baby bring
We are touched to know that life carries on
Around the kitchen we dance and sing

Her parents in awe of what has happened
A miracle, in which they can believe
A new life to cherish, guide and love
A warm welcome to you, baby Eve

Today begins with another trip to the doctor
He is pleased with my progress to date
I've been free from the violent pain so far
I am happy to have it finally abate

Next it is off to visit Doug's salon
For a color and a haircut trim
The day flies by in no time at all
I am entertaining my every whim

Rosie, my friend arrives late in the day
We are going out for dinner and fun
Our favorite musicians are playing in town
We enjoy this treat as the day is done

We head home and chat for quite a while
She is spending the night in our lovely guest room
Her husband and mine are both out of town
It is special to have her here in our home

Our friendship goes back some 20 years ago
When they first joined our musical church group
We were named "Joyful Noise" and that it was
Traveling the state as a singing troupe

Good friendships were made and they remain
Through the many years, we are so very blessed
To have such wonderful people touch our lives
With trust, hope and helping hands put to the test

"A Dream is a Goal With a Deadline"
Napolean Hill

I have been writing for a year and one-half
One book has already been published
I like this idea of dreams and goals
It rates high on my very important list

Sometimes we all are afraid to dream
Believing that we are not deserving
But setting one's dreams into motion
Is freeing, worthwhile and self serving

It is each of us who must set the goal
Nothing is ever really out of reach
With faith, along with the help of God
There is nothing we cannot achieve

Dreams are a sign of looking forward
With glad anticipation of our lives ahead
Our dreams must be nurtured as ourselves
They must remain present and constantly fed

Feeding a dream truly keeps it alive
Anything alive requires much tender care
Treating dreams gently and lovingly
Bathing them in God's beauty and prayer

"You cannot depend on your eyes when your
imagination is out of focus"
Mark Twain

Well, here is a challenge if ever there was
Giving creative energy room to flow
To imagine a thing and believe in it
Is halfway to setting it aglow

We must keep our dreams alive in our hearts
In order to bring them to fruition
Hopes and dreams are the keys it seems
To keeping our minds in good condition

I've been dreaming myself for quite a while
Of a beautiful Labyrinth in the yard
And recently found an octagonal plan
Researching the idea was not very hard

The octagon represents rebirth and renewal
Although most plans are usually round
I'm beginning to actually visualize it complete
And know to walk it will prove most profound

I'm seeing the material take shape already
With wood and plenty of stone
The entire enclosure surrounded by hedges
A place to contemplate and walk alone

"An idea is salvation by imagination"
Frank Lloyd Wright

A new month of summer is here at last
To be creative outside in the sun
How many ideas are floating in a day
We need simply to open up and join in the fun

Go to the park and watch children at play
Their ideas just seem to flow freely
Are we afraid that someone will laugh
If we share our imagination and ideas?

What better way to spend a summer day
To read, make new plans and dream
And then as the day lazily winds down
To stop and enjoy a cone of ice cream

Do you think summer days are better for dreaming
Or is it as simple as being outdoors?
Perhaps just some free time for each of us
From the drudgery of mundane daily chores

"Don't be afraid to take a big step if one is indicated.
You can't cross a chasm in two small steps."
David Lloyd George

I can picture myself afraid at this choice
For I tend to be reserved a bit
But jumping across a large chasm
Can only be done with authentic true grit

How often are we afraid to step out
And take in faith that great leap
It takes quite a bit of courage indeed
And is not for those whose faith is weak

We need but surrender our needless fears
To take full advantage of opportunities given
To live in a continual state of HOPE
Using our talents, which we often keep hidden

To trust in the graces which God bestows
And live our lives to the fullest, free of fear
Takes courage, strength and unwavering faith
To reap the benefits of these blessings so dear

Reach out in faith and take that big step
One's future is patiently waiting to unfold
But taking that first step can sometimes be daunting
Go for it, reach high, have faith and be bold!

About the Author

Lois Vogt Pike began writing poetry and music at the early age of eleven. She is the author of a previous book "Embracing Life – Living With Chronic Pain", also published by iuniverse in 2005. Lois remains active in her local community and is a member of the Litchfield Board of Ethics Commission. She is also the State of CT Representative for the American Pain Foundation (APF) and the American Chronic Pain Association (ACPA). Lois is a member of the Women of the World Steering Committee and has been featured in many news articles. She leads a monthly Support Group for Chronic Pain Sufferers and Caregivers. She is an avid fan of the UCONN Women's Basketball Team. Lois resides with her husband Wilbur L. Pike III, an Organizational Psychologist, in a fully restored farmhouse, which was constructed in 1820, along with their two beloved cats, Ella and Tucker. Her brother, Bert Vogt lives in an attached apartment with his cat Miss Mary. The cover photo shows Lois sitting in the center of a newly constructed 40 ft octagonal Labyrinth, which was built by her husband. It is a wonderful place to walk and meditate, which she does on a daily basis, weather permitting.

www.ingramcontent.com/pod-product-compliance
Lightning Source LLC
Chambersburg PA
CBHW061253280526
45784CB00002B/752